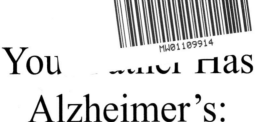

You ~~Mother~~ Has Alzheimer's:

A Primer for Baby Boomers on Dealing *With Our Aging Parents*

Miles Friedman

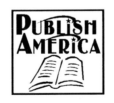

PublishAmerica

Baltimore

© 2002 by Miles Friedman.

All rights reserved. No part of this book may be reproduced in any form without written permission from the publishers, except by a reviewer who may quote brief passages in a review to be printed in a newspaper or magazine.

First printing

ISBN: 1-59129-310-3
PUBLISHED BY PUBLISHAMERICA BOOK
PUBLISHERS
www.publishamerica.com
Baltimore

Printed in the United States of America

Dedication

This book is dedicated to Sol Friedman,
one of the most interesting,
and loved,
people I have ever known.

Acknowledgements

I would like to acknowledge several people who helped make this book possible. I want to thank my wife, Susan Liles Friedman, whose patience and love helped all of us get through my father's illness, and who planted the idea for this book in my head; my children, David and Diana, who gave up lots of free afternoons and evenings to persevere through difficult visits to the nursing home so that they could support their father and be with their grandfather; and my mother-in-law and father-in-law, Lois and Glenn Liles, who made sure that I knew I would always have their support.

There are two other individuals who need to be mentioned for their contributions: Wilkie Leith, whose editing and constructive criticism helped make me seem more articulate than would otherwise have been the case; and Buck Waters, whose encouragement and unflagging support helped bring me to this point.

Alan, perhaps this will help Dad live on for all of us.

Preface: Did They Say, "Alzheimer's?"

"Mr. Friedman, your father has Alzheimer's." That would have been amongst the worst news I'd ever had, except that no one ever really said those words in just that way. The doctor didn't really tell me that my father had Alzheimer's. In fact, the doctor did tell me that when dealing with Alzheimer's Disease no doctor is in a position to make a definitive diagnosis. I'm told that the only way to make a definite confirmation of Alzheimer's is through an autopsy. Most of us are reluctant to authorize an autopsy for a living relative.

Alzheimer's is a slippery, black hole disease, with more unknown factors than known. For the growing number of us who must cope with our mothers and fathers falling prey to this terror, no primer we read can help us deal with our degenerating loved ones. I found that my first experience involved a startling realization of how many questions I had and finding that no one had any satisfying answers.

This book is largely about the confusion brought on by Alzheimer's, for our infected relatives, and for those of us who must look after them. More than that, I have realized that many of the issues I had to deal with were common to my other baby boomer friends whose parents were beginning to lose their ability to function independently in the world. The doctors call it "dementia". Those same doctors tell us that there are many causes, which include but are not limited to, Alzheimer's.

This started out to be a book specifically about dealing with parents who suffer from Alzheimer's, but has become something more. In the process of pulling my thoughts together for the book, I realized that many of the things that belong here, also apply to many of the other aging parents and their adult children who are bewildered about how to handle them. My experiences with Dad led several other people in my office to seek advice from me, as they dealt with aging parents, especially in cases where those parents were not living in the same town as their offspring. Together, we realized that these families were going through many of the same challenges that we went through, concerning living accommodations, health and security issues, finances and legal arrangements, and none of the other parents had Alzheimer's. There are those who believe that doctors are now putting the Alzheimer's name to what were once thought of as generic aging symptoms, thereby accounting for the growing number of patients with this diagnosis. Others feel that Alzheimer's is simply one of the many forms and causes of dementia, which, to some extent, is an unavoidable consequence of aging. In any event, there are lots of parents of baby boomers, who are living longer, and losing the degree of control over their lives that they, and we, would like them to have.

This is not to say that Alzheimer's and other forms of dementia are indistinguishable from the normal aging process. In fact, I have encountered some of the differences. An aging parent might get off a plane and would have already forgotten what he had been served for lunch a scant hour ago, while the Alzheimer's sufferer, might, immediately upon arrival, be wondering why he was in an airport, or even what an airport was. However, even given stark differences in the degree and kind of confusion that Alzheimer's creates, there are lots of conditions in between that disease and normal forgetfulness, which generate similar kinds of problems for us as concerned offspring. There are other medical conditions, such as small strokes, and chemical imbalances, sometimes caused by medications, that can leave our parents confused. Environmental factors, such as a recent move away from a familiar home or the death of a loved one, can disorient an aging parent. Some of these have only temporary effects, others are more permanent, but all can lead to the kind of abject confusion that might be called dementia, as opposed to the relatively benign loss of short-term memory that comes naturally with age. In all cases, we are dealing with these forces that act upon our elderly parents in ways that none of us could have predicted.

We are the sandwich generation...the baby boom success stories whose worlds become more challenging as we are forced to deal with aging parents and growing children, with both generations depending heavily upon us for their well being. No matter how well adjusted we might think we are, dealing with our parents and our children is a heavy responsibility, and one that often confronts us in a way that leaves us with little time to pay attention to our own frailties and neuroses.

If you are one of the bewildered souls who is trying to maintain the quality of life for your aging loved ones - loved ones who once guided your life and now cannot survive without you - then this book is for you. This is not a book simply about the decline and fall of my Dad, though that is one inescapable element of the story. Writing this book has allowed me a certain amount of reflection upon the relationship I enjoyed with my father, and what that says about who he was and how we both coped with his descent into oblivion.

This is a book about the decisions you must make that will affect the life of your infected loved one, and about his confusion and yours, as you struggle to figure out what he knows and what he does not and what he can do for himself and what he can't and what you can trust him to do for himself and what you can't. The book is about everything from making sure he gets his medication to establishing ground rules for determining where he lives and for insuring that his finances will be protected.

This book is not a medical treatise on the science of Alzheimer's; but rather a layman's book on how I learned about the pain of dealing with an aging and increasingly confused parent, and how I learned about those who can help you, those who will hurt you, and those who could care less. The book is about dealing with a divided medical community, a confusing government labyrinth and a host of charlatans and thieves who view your parents as their livelihood.

I can offer no definitive answers, only a series of experiences, impressions and recommendations. Perhaps the book will help you to at least know what questions to ask, and where you might find some of the answers. I offer this book as a loving tribute to my father and his valiant fight to preserve his dignity, and as a source of information and reassurance to those, like me, who must go through this process without a clue as to what our parents "dementia" is all about.

As I try to look at the big picture, it seems to me that one can break down the areas of uncertainty into several categories. In no particular order, these are:

· Health: Is my father all right, and is there something more I can be doing to make sure he is all right for as long as possible? Are we doing everything we can? Is there a treatment for Alzheimer's and what should my expectations be?

· Living Arrangements: How long can my father live on his own, and when he cannot, what are his options and his optimal situation? What standards do I use to determine a safe level of self-sufficiency and how much do his surroundings affect his well- being?

· Finances and Legal Arrangements: Has my father made reasonable arrangements to secure his financial future, even if that means living in a nursing home; and, how long can he continue to manage his own money? How can I help when I don't want to interfere? What are his rights and my rights?

· Sources of Help: Where can I turn for advice, comfort, assistance with my father's needs, legal and financial counsel, etc.? How can the government help and what must I be careful about, to avoid running afoul of the government?

Safety and Sanity: What concerns should I have about my father's behavior and the way it affects his own well being and that of others? How should I act toward him and what should I tell others? How long can he go on driving?

This book is written to reflect what my life felt like during my father's struggle with Alzheimer's. Life became a swirling mix of remembrances, rudely interrupted by the harsh reality of Dad's degeneration. I managed to hang on to, and even to relive many happy childhood memories, and somehow, those memories helped me cope.

Each chapter begins with one of my most vivid remembrances, and concludes with a narrative about the Alzheimer's years. In the sections dealing with the Alzheimer's "present", I have included advice on how to address the challenges we confronted.

Chapter One

Didn't That Used to be Cary Grant?

Rockland County, New York, November 1966: Let's Roll the Videotape

I knew that my father had brought home a huge box the night before, and woke expectantly that morning like a kid at Christmas. My father had just picked up his new videotape recorder late the previous night, with the promise that we would all set up and try out the glorious new machine together. We still called them videotape recorders back in the early 1960s, before they were VCRs or camcorders or multimedia electronics. That year Sony came out with the first machine that could record and play back using reel-to-reel videotape. All at once this modern technology, the tape machine, threatened to replace the home movie camera and provide a means for recording your favorite TV show when you were not able to watch it.

My father called out my name in a stage whisper. He was hurrying down the hallway past my bedroom. I caught a glimpse of his shorty pajamas and terry cloth robe whizzing by my door and realized that, teenager or not, I would have to move fast if I was going to catch him downstairs before all of the goods were out of the box. We were opening, not only the first videotape machine that our family had owned, but the first home video machine that any one in our county would own, because my father had made arrangements with our local electronics store to sell us the first one.

I bounded down the stairs of our split-level ranch zipping up my jeans and straightening my tee shirt - some things we must do, no matter how excited - only to hear the sound of a sharp Stanley knife already slicing through the packing tape on the huge box. As I hit the floor running, my father looked up with his trademark look of glee, a sly grin spreading across his face. The box was so big, it took up most of our pool table, and before I knew it, the rest of the pool table was covered with documents and cables. I sat down next to my dad, almost as thrilled as he was. We were preparing to crack open a technological miracle that would change our lives, and those of most Americans, forever. It was like sharing Christmas morning with a thoroughly delighted child, a joy that I have since shared with my own children, many times.

I noticed through the sliding glass doors that snow was falling, gently on the unraked leaves of the backyard. My father had been too preoccupied to rake leaves, and I had been too lazy. Beyond the white flakes that were settling on our multi-hued yard, a slim crust of ice was forming, like pudding skin, on the little manmade lake we lived on. My father had eyes only for the box and the contents, although every once in a while he snuck a glance at me to see if I was as excited as he was.

I knew that my father had always been an electronics buff. I had the rare pleasure of being the son of a man who invented electronic toys for a living. I also knew that my father had been trained as an electrical engineer, though I had seen this mostly through his inventions and his capacity with televisions and stereo equipment. Dad always treasured his toys, as do I. He read the trade journals and magazines religiously and always stayed on top of the latest technologies, both for professional purposes and for recreational uses. He had been following the development of home videotape equipment for quite some time and as the shipment of Sony's first consumer models approached he was beside himself with excitement.

Videotape has a huge advantage over conventional film because it is instantaneous; like taking a Polaroid picture, it needs no developing. We have all come to love this latest development in instant gratification, as we follow our kids around with the camcorder and immediately replay the tape. Videotape also works well for television because it delivers, somehow, a more intimate and lifelike experience than movie film.

I think Dad saw the invention of home videotape machines as the most revolutionary event in consumer electronics since the invention of television. He was determined to have one at the first possible moment. Over the years, my father had done quite a bit of business with a fine local electronics retailer, from whom he purchased things like transistors that he used in his work and stereo equipment for his teenage sons. My father convinced Henry, the owner of the shop, to order a few of the Sony machines, which were not considered to be a lock of any kind for retail success. I believe Henry ordered six of the new inventions from his wholesaler, but promised my father the very first one. In return, Dad agreed to open and experiment with the machine immediately. Henry would not have to take a chance on selling the newfangled thing to any of his other regular customers until Dad had proven that the newfangled machine could work.

Dad reveled in his role of pioneer, not only getting to play with a great new toy, but to be a part of history by trying that first videotape machine out. Henry's store would be, for some time, the only place in our town where one could buy these videotape machines, and my father's technical expertise and considerable trade with Henry were the main reasons Henry had agreed to take a chance. This, along with some of my father's revolutionary toy designs, was a means for him to play a role in the history of electronics. He may not have invented the home videotape machine, but he certainly helped bring it to the consumers of Rockland County, New York.

As I watched the bits and pieces of consumer electronics history come out of the massive box, I wondered what in the world this machine could do to have my father so excited. What ultimately arose from that box was an enormous piece of equipment, the size of a professional caliber reel-to-reel audio tape recorder. It had cables as thick as your fingers and an impressive AC adaptor to plug into the wall. These original machines had to be connected to a television to record, because they basically took the viewing image off the TV and recorded it. My father of course, knew all this and was prepared. He had purchased a small black and white Sony television - the magical machine would only record in black and white...which was OK, since that is how most TV shows were recorded - and a rolling stand to house all of the equipment. My Dad was ready for home videotaping!

By now my brother, Alan – age nine - had wandered, sleepily, downstairs, but, according to my father's instructions, my mother was not to be disturbed until the machine was set up and proven to work. She had been skeptical, but totally supportive, as was usually the case. My brother and I had charge of the instruction manuals, which was no small task, as they approached the size and heft of the encyclopedia (you know, when they used to be on books, not CD ROM). As my father connected each cable our collective excitement grew. Finally, all the connections appeared to have been made, but before we could hit the all-important Power button, my mother quietly slipped into the room. My father was unfazed, and warned her that we were flying blind. He gave her the honor of hitting the power button for the first time.

The machine hummed to life, we all applauded, and my father picked up the massive camera, which of course was separate from the main machine and connected by one of those snake-thick cables. As we watched, just minutes later, and saw our first instant home movies, I simply shook my head and thought to myself that truly, my father was a genius. Shortly thereafter, we tried recording from the television set, which also worked splendidly. We spent the entire day playing with that machine, with the highlight being a series of recordings my father and his best friend made, in which they dubbed in their own dialogue to a movie recorded from the TV. Most of our neighbors passed through the house at one time or another that day, confirming what I already knew and had thought early that morning: that my Dad was brilliant, a true electronics genius.

Fairfax County, Virginia, 1996: Why is the Screen Blue?

Thirty years later, I was watching my father sit in his nursing home room, fiddling with his combination TV/VCR, trying to get the screen to change from all blue to something with pictures. He had no clue.

"Is this thing supposed to just be blue all the time? I thought it was supposed to show pictures," he said.

"Yes, Dad, the VCR is built in. You're not on a channel, so there's no TV show coming in, but if you hit Play, the movie will start".

He said he understood and went on pushing and pulling buttons, with no result. He did not want me to touch the controls, and snatched the remote away when I tried to do an end run with that. I was surprised and pleased that he even understood what the remote could do. Finally, while I distracted him, a nurse who had come in to check on him, managed to hit the right button, and the Cary Grant movie came on, prompting immediate and genuine, though non-comprehending, laughter from my father.

We sat within touching distance of each other in the cramped nursing home room. I was on Dad's bed, and Dad sat in a non-descript armchair. On the other side of the green curtain an elderly man from Viet Nam coughed without enthusiasm. Mr. Ky never said much, though this may have been because his English was not good. The room had a faintly antiseptic smell, and was bathed in a gray light that could have signaled any time of day and any season of the year.

I tried to understand how Dad had ever gotten this bad...to remember what he had been like in recent years and how quickly he had degenerated. As he chuckled along with Cary Grant, I tried to reconcile the father who had been an electronics genius with the man who could not hit the play button on a VCR.

He surprised me for a moment, a pleasant surprise, "Say...didn't that used to be Cary Grant"? My father would say. "Is he still alive or what...I bet he's dead." my father concluded, before I could answer either question. I didn't have to answer, because he had already forgotten the question.

This was not unusual. My father would be given to occasional flashes of insight, some mundane, and others fairly clever. There was no predicting, especially at this more advanced stage, what he would and would not remember or understand. Sometimes he knew me, and sometimes he did not, and this could vary even during the same visit.

As these moments so often did, the incident got me started thinking about how all this began and where our adventure in Alzheimer's had taken us. Once again, conventional thinking would not do, as Alzheimer's stories have no defined beginning, even medical science is vague on this subject. Yet we can all look back and try to decide when we at least realized that we were dealing with the dreaded disease and all of its implications.

I was sad to see Dad so confused and non-comprehending, and sorry for myself and for the loss of a father who I had always looked to for advice and guidance. Self-pity seemed to be a bit of an indulgence, when my father was the one who was ill. Still, once your father has progressed to the nursing home stage, the real burden is on those around him, as his needs are mostly taken care of.

But what lies in between; what is the transition like from competent human being to disoriented nursing home patient?

From Forgetfulness to Alzheimer's...

My father had always had a bad memory; in fact, he had always had an appalling lack of memory, a fact that some researchers now would find significant. I heard on Good Morning America that many Alzheimer's patients are, not surprisingly, people who had long histories of forgetfulness. This is, however, deceptive, as being forgetful is not, in itself, a predictor of future Alzheimer's, so don't panic. What's more, science tells us that there are numerous causes of forgetfulness, including the natural process of aging. My understanding is that the studies have focused on individuals with particularly long and egregious memory problems, not mere forgetfulness.

Ah, but where does that magic line exist? We all suffer the

frustration of a loved one, not always a parent, who never seems to remember anything. My own wife would tell you that she never tells me anything because I just will forget what she says, anyway. You can probably imagine what I'm talking about: what we are doing Saturday night; the name of my son's math teacher; the name of the man she hired to cut down some trees, the day he is coming and the trees we plan to cut down.

I can instigate a heated discussion with something like, "Honey, did we ever decide what to do about those trees that are overhanging the house?"

A perfectly natural question, if only she hadn't told me just two days before about the man coming on Saturday to cut the trees down. Of course it riles her to know that I can still tell her who pitched every game of the 1960 World Series and can identify the leading batters in both the American and National Leagues that same year! This might all be cause for concern, since Alzheimer's can, indeed begin with such selective memory lapses, and the disease is often characterized by short-term memory loss. Fortunately, or unfortunately, depending upon your point of view, I have heard the same complaint from more wives than I could list if I took the rest of the chapter. In fact, I work in an office with four married women, each of whom would swear that her husband would forget whether he was wearing pants if he did not look down periodically!

I don't mean to make light of a frightening phenomenon, only to illustrate a point. Memory is a relative thing, and not a good indicator of medical conditions, at least not to the amateur diagnostician. On the other hand, my father's memory lapses were legendary. For example, I had a high school friend who lived a block away, and visited my house every day for six years, usually at dinnertime. My father was extremely fond of this friend, as was my mother, and they saw him almost every day. At our high school graduation party my father still was stumbling over my friend's name, checking with me to see whether he had the right guy. It was not as though Jack - I kid you not - was a tough name to remember.

The stories go on. During my first visit home from college, I had called my high school girlfriend, though we had, by then gone our separate ways, to get together. My mother asked that we come back to the house so she could say hello and catch up with Joan, since she had been part of our household for nearly four years, and grown quite close to my entire family. Much to my relief, Dad remembered her name. Unfortunately, he could not recall whether we were still together, or whether she had gone on to attend the same college that I did. In fact, we had gone to school in separate cities, and it had been a major bone of contention during our entire senior year.

I remember sitting in a bar with friends from my hometown several years later, in 1972, and wondering out loud whether my father could already be suffering from senility at the relatively young age of fifty. That night he had forgotten what kind of car I drove, who I was dating at the time, and where my favorite restaurant was.

Don't get me wrong...this is not about my father having a mental block toward everything that I did. He had always taken a great interest in my life, and we had always shared a great deal with each other. I merely cite my own frustrations with his infamous memory, although my mother was the one who could have filled an encyclopedia with tales of unbelievable memory lapses by Dad, almost since the day they met. She, for her part, chalked it up to his being a creative genius with a streak of eccentricity. After all, he invented toys for a living, read every piece of science fiction literature ever written and spent much of his time dreaming of far off worlds, and impossible inventions. He was, to our family, and many who knew him, sort of our own version of the eccentric genius, Dr. Brown, played by Christopher Lloyd in the Back to the Future movies.

Thus, we wrote off a lot of Dad's memory failures. Do I believe that this was a portent of more ominous things? Maybe...and maybe not. Dad did have a terrible memory, and he did, eventually, develop Alzheimer's. This is not scientific evidence, merely an anecdotal history.

The question posed here is: When did we first suspect that forgetfulness had turned into disease?

It is still hard, even in retrospect, to say. My mother died in 1982, after a long and miserable battle with an inoperable tumor. My father remarried shortly thereafter, and was quite happy for a time, until his second wife developed a debilitating disease that haunted both of them for several years. When she died ten years after my mother, my father seemed to go down hill, in many ways. The most startling change was the degradation of his memory, and to a lesser extent, his cognitive abilities in general. Dad went back to Florida after the funeral, to the house where both of his wives had died. He had done the same thing shortly after he lost my mother, and had seemed to restore something of a normal life. My brother and I did the best we could to monitor him from Virginia, with almost daily phone calls and bimonthly visits from one or the other of us. He also had friends and some family close by, and we stayed in touch with them, as well, as an extra check.

By 1993, when Dad was 70, we had become concerned that he was not bouncing back any faster, but were still convinced that his tumultuous, heart rending battle to save two wives, both of whom literally died in his arms after years of misery, had taken a toll. Dad seemed to be of relatively good spirits, and was once again trying to find someone to date, which encouraged everyone. By later that year he had a new girlfriend, a darling woman who had lost her husband of 45 years and was finding great comfort in my father. She was truly a tonic to Dad, as his spirits rose and his ambitions about life lifted too.

I visited Dad in the fall of 1993 and spent the weekend at his house in Ft. Lauderdale, before driving up to Palm Beach for a work-related conference. After visiting Dad I was in high spirits at the thought of how well he was doing. We had gone out several times with his "friend" Annie, and had the kind of fun you do when going out with a couple of old college buddies...well, maybe not as wild – of course we still had to listen to tapes of Henry Mancini in the Cadillac and ate every dinner by four o'clock. But certainly we had enjoyed very entertaining and amusing outings. Clearly, they were very much in love. He had definitely filled a void of loneliness in her life, and she was certainly bringing a sense of stability and normalcy back into his life. He seemed really, grounded, for lack of a better word. His entire perspective on life had returned.

Even the time that Dad and I spent together, just the two of us was different in a positive way. He had his sense of humor back - well...it was a sense of humor only in the loosest sense, the kind that found laughter in the name Lewis Boles, because of its resemblance to the term, loose bowels - and we talked and laughed late into each night. We also talked openly and warmly about our past together, our family and even about things we had once disagreed on. These were powerful conversations...discussions that renewed the bonds between us and restored much of my father's fatherly image. I felt more kinship, than sympathy for him at this time, which seemed to be the way things should be between father and son. I realized that I was happy for Dad, but also happy for me. I felt as though I had my father back.

I visited again in early 1994 and found that the romantic bliss between Dad and Annie continued. The only quarrel between them was over whether to marry or not. He, like most men, was eager to marry, but she was not. My Dad wanted the whole deal, marriage, live together in his house, visit his and her grandchildren together, etc. For Annie, the whole picture was perfect, except she just wanted to spend time together, while maintaining separate residences, and to an extent, separate identities. They would work it out...I was sure.

What concerned me a little more were Annie's complaints about Dad's forgetfulness. Most of it sounded all too familiar, some the usual complaints that women had about their men, some of her stories sounding like a lifetime of dealing with my Dad. Annie was insistent, however, that his memory lapses went beyond the comprehensible, and were worsening at an alarming rate. He would forget about toast he put in the toaster; he would forget that he had left the TV on; he would forget what time they were supposed to get together; he would forget where he parked his car; and so the complaints went.

I noticed that, when we talked, Dad had forgotten little bits of history that were fairly significant, such as when my mother died, who he was married to during certain years in the late 1970s and early 1980s and which wife he had taken on various trips. This frustrated and concerned me, particularly when we quarreled over what month and year my mother died. Annie believed me, and said that this was par for the course. She asked what I thought about taking him to the doctor. He was seeing his family physician, who still assured him that his mental lapses were the result of mental blockages, caused by all the pain and anguish he had suffered. This explanation seemed to make sense, but Annie was not convinced, and we agreed to stay in touch on this. Perhaps we just wanted this rationale to be true.

That summer, Dad and Annie came to visit us in Virginia, and my concerns grew as a result of that visit. The concern began when my son, David, then ten, and I picked them up at the airport, and I asked Dad how his trip had been. His reply was, "What trip?" During that same visit Dad had trouble remembering which of his wives was my mother.

One particularly warm afternoon we were watching the kids play Frisbee in my backyard. Dad and Annie seemed happy to be with us, and my wife Susan was talking to Annie, who she liked immensely. Birds chirped and swooped around us, enriching the air with their sweet songs. Buzzing bees capped the flowers that ringed the yard and the aroma of Virginia in June filled our senses. I could almost imagine being a kid again, playing in my own backyard, while my Dad watched. David and Diana, my children, ten and seven, were laughing loudly, and showing off for my Dad and Annie.

Without warning, a discordant note sounded, innocent – and not – all at the same time. Dad smiled warmly, winked at me, and commented on how talented his grandchildren were. Then he leaned in close, as if to share a secret, and asked me who owned the park we were playing in.

I laughed, thinking he was making a joke, but then the puzzlement in his eyes showed me that this was no joke. I was a bit angry with Dad for being so stupid, and at once I realized that I was also embarrassed by his question. The last thing that I was thinking about was the implication for my father's health or his state of mind. There would be plenty of time for that, and by that evening I did begin to wonder what was happening to my father.

There were still conflicting bits of evidence. During that same visit, Dad taught my seven year old daughter, Diana, how to play chess, showed David how to improve his pitching motion and gave Susan his recipe for potato pancakes. He and Annie seemed happier than ever. The look in their eyes and the doting way they had with each other reminded me of my parents when they were younger, and gave me a sense of peace about their lives together. Annie had taken Dad to another doctor, who felt that the memory problems and even a certain level of confusion were plausibly explained by the extraordinary circumstances of suffering the lingering deaths of two wives. He suggested giving it some time. We were to watch him closely for any changes.

By January 1995 Dad's memory seemed to be worsening, and Annie had threatened to stop seeing him if he would not find a doctor who could help him. Dad was standing by the diagnosis of the two doctors he had seen and claimed to "just be a little more forgetful than usual". He had been fighting a series of colds and sore throats, and blamed cold medication for any additional memory problems. Annie was concerned; I was checking in almost daily, and had planned to go down to Florida in early February.

Just a few weeks before my planned visit, we were having one of the February snow storms that can catch the Washington area by surprise, since big storms are rare, and the weatherman never predicts them. Susan and I were watching the wintry scene through our den window, and enjoying the warmth of the fire in our woodstove, when the phone rang; it was Annie, and she was nearly hysterical.

"Your father's been in a car accident; he's in the hospital," Annie forced out, breathlessly. I repeated what she had said, and could see the look of alarm in Susan's face.

"Is he all right; what happened?" I managed to say.

He was all right from the accident, but had apparently passed out in the car and hit a guardrail.

"Miles, it's awful. Your Dad didn't even know who he was or

where he lived when the police found him. "

Dad had remembered who Annie was and had given the police her phone number. As far as she could tell, he had been forgetting to take antibiotics that the doctor had given him for strep throat, had become feverish and overheated, had fainted from having an extremely high temperature, and had hit the guardrail before coming to a stop.

I went cold. Despite Annie's assurances that the accident had been minor, there was no hiding the panic in her voice. The disorientation that had caused the accident, and had continued afterwards, had badly unnerved her. I promised Annie that I would call Dad at the hospital and get back to her. I could not dial the phone fast enough. I think part of what had me so upset was the fear that I had taken Dad's forgetfulness too lightly, had made excuses, and had dangerously overlooked the signs of trouble.

When I called Dad at the hospital, he seemed back to his old self, and the forgotten antibiotics, resulting fever, etc. all seemed plausible. But a call back to Annie made me realize that she was not convinced. I can still remember her saying, "You must come down here and see him for yourself...something is not right with him, and I am at my wit's end. Please, please, please come down and spend some time. You will see what I mean."

So...maybe it was that late night phone call from Annie, or maybe it was the car accident itself in January 1995 that brought me to the conclusion that there was something more than bad memory and mental anguish affecting my father. Hearing Annie so upset got to me. She had seemed upset out of proportion to what had happened in the car. Annie was now convinced that my Dad had some kind of mental impairment. Her pleas convinced me that it was time to get more involved. I could not have ignored her.

Susan took me to the airport the next morning, and, as always, I marveled at her skill in weaving her way around and through heavy Washington traffic. This trip to Florida to see Dad was not going to be like the many idyllic family car trips we had taken so many years ago.

Chapter Two

Why Are All the Cars Going the Other Way?

The Catskills, New York State, 1959: Bingo in the Dining Hall at
Eight O'clock

The new Pontiac rounded the curve on Route 17 at speed, as
though the twisting road were as straight as an arrow, bringing the
mountain view into our line of sight faster than usual. The
breathtaking view only served to heighten the excitement that always
accompanied our trip to the Catskill Mountains, just north of New
York City, each summer. The sun seemed brighter than ever, the
mountains higher, the trees greener than they had any right to be. Far
below, past the guardrail, some lazy loop of water meandered through
large gray boulders, and even the boulders looked wonderful to me.
I marveled at how well the new car rode, and at the consummate
skill with which my father piloted his pride and joy through the
twisting mountain road. Everything was right with the world: new
car, beautiful day, baby brother sleeping quietly, my folks chatting
amiably in the front seat, interrupted periodically by my mother's
admonitions to "slow down a little, for goodness sake!" and two
weeks of heaven in the Catskills now, literally, right around the corner.

I am proud of my New York City roots, but not foolish enough to
let nostalgia convince me that I enjoyed spending my summers in
the Bronx. I lived, fifty weeks each year, for the two-week hiatus in
the mountains, and everything that such trips always involved. New
York was an experience for a kid, a cauldron of activity, a hotbed of
first-rate professional sports, a cultural Mecca and a true melting
pot that exposed you to multiple ethnic and cultural experiences.

The Bronx, my part of New York City, was also hot, covered with asphalt, busy with traffic, noisy and smelly, and in no small way, a relatively dangerous place to grow up. Most of those dangers were not life threatening unless you count the number of times we came within inches of death on the grilles of cars who insisted on driving through our stickball fields, which their drivers seemed to think were city streets. But there were constant reminders that life could be perilous, even in the 1950s. There was the time that five kids, neither friends nor enemies of mine, decided to make me the subject of a science experiment. They each held large chunks of dry ice, given them by the driver of the ice dream truck, and they desperately needed to understand why he had told them not to touch the ice, making them hold their treats in ice cream wrappers, instead. They held me down and applied dry ice to my face, until one of the kids realized that a large, bright red welt was developing along my cheek. Fortunately, the doctors were wrong; the searing burn from the dry ice left no permanent scar. The police were called and they visited each of the kids, but no one, to my knowledge, has ever been prosecuted in New York City for a dry ice attack.

Being a kid, living in the bowels of a large city had its simple limitations. We managed to play ball, sure. We had stickball, and a wide variety of other, more unusual, baseball substitutes, all played with what was then known as a Spaulding High Bouncer, the hardest, purest rubber balls ever made, with a rough, dark skin, rather than the smooth, pink skin of the other most popular rubber ball of our day. We played punch ball, slap ball, stoop ball, wall ball and so on...all named for the method in which the ball was hit by the person at home plate. For the record, you either hit the ball with your hand, or bounced the ball hard off the stoop, wall or other inanimate object. Our playing fields varied, though none were completely satisfactory. The safest was the sidewalk, which worked well, until a building superintendent chased us. This made for a long, but extremely narrow field of play, which encouraged both power AND accuracy, traits that would serve any hitter well, if indeed, these games would translate into baseball prowess.

Other games were played totally in the street, which was wider and made for less harassment, unless you count the cars. At least you could see the cars coming in this game. More unpredictable, were the games we played that situated home plate on one sidewalk and placed the bases on the opposite sidewalk, requiring the batter to run across the street to round the bases. This game was, in some ways, the most exciting, for reasons that had little to do with baseball.

We had parks and playgrounds, of course, but these had their limitations. You would have to make arrangements to get to a place to play, and organize thoroughly to insure a critical mass of players. Then there were the travel hazards. One park, a mere fifteen-minute walk from my apartment building, was known territory of a group of "other kids". Nothing so ominous or romantic as an organized gang, just the "other kids". You really did not want to mess with these "other kids", although I must admit that the worst thing they ever did to me was to make my little group of friends play with them in a marathon baseball game that lasted some seven hours and made all of us miss our appointed time to be home. The other travel hazard tended to be found in the form of dangerous neighborhoods that might be gang turfs, en route to a park or playground. There were recognized turfs that you stayed away from, and then there were the ad hoc groups that could arise on any given day. I know for a fact that my good friend, Richard, was chased and generally roughed up on every single day of every single summer, until he went off to college. Unfortunately for Richard, he had to cross the imaginary line that separated 198th street from 199th street to get to my house. He never even questioned the daily beatings.

The annual trip to the Catskills was my escape to nirvana. Two weeks in the Catskills meant sleeping in a bungalow - a cabin - with open windows, and birds chirping. The Catskills meant evenings strolling through the trees, listening to the sound of the wind, and the voices of singing and laughing grownups coming through the screens on the main building where the entertainment played. The trip to the mountains meant playing real baseball at least once every day, and having several pickup games of whiffle ball in between. It was swimming in the pool, collecting salamanders from under rocks and alongside the road, picking blueberries - which to my surprise did not come from a can - rolling in the grass for no particular reason, and swinging idly in a hammock with a book in my hand, and no cares in my head.

Every trip to the Catskills includes mental footage of my father, who I spent most of every day with. He played whiffle ball with me, my friends and my brother at least once each day, and taught me his wicked underhand curve that later served me so well during my years of playing intramural softball in college and graduate school. He flew kites with me, almost every day, usually early in the morning, when Alan and my mother were still asleep in the bungalow, showing me how to get those red and blue paper triangles aloft, even when the wind was little more than a whisper. Dad helped me make my first lizard lounge, just as I would do with my own son years later, using a shoebox lined with foil or something. We always planned to let the little guys go back to the wild after a day or two, a moot point, as most managed to make daring escapes during their first night. These were the most exotic pets I could imagine, and their colors and behavior thrilled me. I always marveled at the delicacy with which my father's thick hands held those tiny creatures.

On one memorable trip to the Catskills my father also taught me to play bridge. Tired of poker and blackjack, I had begged to learn more challenging card games. During the summer of 1958, my father had taught his eight-year-old son the game that I enjoy to this day. Now he did have a pragmatic reason for this: while most of the escapees from the city sat around playing mah jong, canasta - mostly the women - or poker and gin - mostly the men - there were still always a loyal group that would search for a bridge game. And, of course, card games in the Catskills, as required by ancient custom, were always played for money, generally small change, though not always. Who would have thought that the kind, pudgy, nice looking man in the glasses and his cute little kid could make for serious competition in a game as sophisticated as bridge? Well...the people who often lost as much as two or three whole dollars in just a single afternoon, found out the hard way.

There must be a touch of larceny in our family. That same sneaky tactic was employed by my grandmother, who taught me a card game called, casino, a close cousin of five hundred rummy, at which she and I routinely took on bevies of white haired old ladies, who never stopped chortling over how cute I was, as we cleaned their clocks and emptied their flowered change purses.

That, and more, is what I thought about as our new Pontiac rounded the bend, and my father said, as he always did at this spot, "Well, we're in the home stretch. It won't be long now!" The car rounded the curve and our precious little bungalow colony, owned by my mother's childhood friend, came into view.

There amidst the trees it sat, a ramshackle collection of old wooden buildings…my Shangri La. Dominating them all was a large central building that was the dining room, meeting and games room and entertainment hall. To the rear of the building was the hot, poorly ventilated kitchen, which sat in stark contrast to the relatively large screened porch at the front, a porch that was liberally dotted with rockers and gliders. Surrounding the main building were a dozen or so bungalows, which we would now call cabins, except they weren't so fancy. They all had a couple of small bedrooms, a single bathroom and a screened porch in front. The only TV antenna was on the main building, so you did not watch a whole lot of television, which was also a nice break from my normal routine.

But the humble buildings only told part of the story. The whole ensemble was carefully ensconced in a beautiful woodland setting that Walt Disney would have been proud to sketch. Giant trees lined the gravel drive, and their huge green leaves neatly camouflaged the cabins. A constant chorus of chirping birds and buzzing insects played their lovely background music, adding to the idyllic setting. Joyful vacationers, freed temporarily from the bonds of New York City, strolled through the grounds, talking and laughing, without a care in the world. For good measure, the proverbial babbling stream meandered casually along in front of the place, and wound its way through grounds. An old canvas hammock hung invitingly between two massive oaks, and massive wooden deck chairs dotted the landscape.

In 1959 my father designed and installed the first sound system they had ever had at the bungalow colony, allowing them to pipe music throughout the complex. My own favorite was the score from South Pacific. The owners could also now make critical announcements that could reach all the guests at once, such as, "Tonight's bingo game has been moved back from 7 p.m. to 8 p.m. to allow everyone a little extra time to digest tonight's dinner!" For a solid week, Dad labored over that sound system, which he managed to keep under the owner's very meager budget. The sound system worked perfectly on test day, and at dinner, they all applauded my father and proclaimed him a genius.

We got in the car only on seldom trips into the tiny town nearby, whose main attraction for me, was the fabulous pinball machine in the candy store at the top of the hill. Otherwise, stepping into the car would mean the dreaded day when we would be going back to the city. For five years I threw up in the car on every one of those trips home.

Years later a ride in the car with my father was to induce nausea again, for much different reasons.

Broward County, Florida 1995: But This Lane Puts Me Closer to My Left Turn

It only took a second for my brother and me to realize that we were not in a turning lane. Clearly, my father had moved into a lane that would soon include the excitement of oncoming traffic. Alan and I had decided on this visit to give my father a chance to prove that he really was OK to drive. I watched from the back seat, as my brother tried to wrestle the wheel away from my father, who protested that we were crazy, and that we were going to get us all killed. He was quite sure that it was all right to be in this lane, especially as it was shorter to turn left from this lane. This was no country road, but a two lane state highway, with no divider.

Somehow, with my pleas from the backseat added to the commotion, my father allowed my brother to steer us back onto the right shoulder and he braked to a stop. Upon calm reflection, he admitted that he had gotten a little confused, citing the fact that construction had changed the roadway just recently - he was right about that. He was calm, logical, and persuasive, and almost got us to believe him. He yielded control of the vehicle to my brother, and continued to speak reasonably from the front passenger's seat, explaining how massive changes in the local roads and highways were to blame for his bouts with dislocation behind the wheel, which Annie had told us about.

This was, in effect, our first family lesson in dealing with Alzheimer's: the patient doesn't realize what's happening for a long time, when he/she does, they do not want to acknowledge or accept it, and they are quite capable, whatever mental failings they may have, of making a vehement case for letting them go about their business. Don't be fooled. We were very lucky that my father did not kill someone during those final months he had been driving. After that night, which was his road test with us, we made sure that he never drove again.

My father had not only driven on the wrong side of the road, he had driven with great hesitancy, had speeded up and slowed down at apparently random moments, and had gotten lost in his own housing development. The signs had been there for some time, but he was still getting around, albeit fitfully. Annie had described his growing bouts of disorientation behind the wheel. Yet, he had always gotten them home at night; in fact, he drove more assuredly with her by his side, and had been staying out of trouble until his one-man fender bender. It was the look in his eyes while driving, a look that I could not miss from the backseat as it reflected in the rearview mirror, which convinced me. He had no grasp of what was happening...almost the way I feel when playing a particularly tough video game for the first time. The kids know that look on my face, vague recognition, without any confidence. My son will get aggravated and say, "Dad, it's not like you have never played a video game before. You just have to figure it out!"

That is what I thought about my father that night, "It's not like he's never driven before. He has an impeccable driving record dating back over fifty years." He would remind us of that, with passion, as he argued his fitness to drive over the coming days and months. In fact, he did not give up on the idea of driving until he reached a stage so advanced that he had little idea what a car was.

We spent almost a week in Florida with Dad and Annie. Several things stood out about Dad and his condition. He was far more lucid and in control of his environment when he was with Annie, and especially when he was at her condo with her. He had spent little time alone in recent months and had barely lived in his own condo. Dad had sold his house six months earlier, and though he lived in the same housing development, the apartment was relatively unfamiliar territory. In fact, he had barely unpacked. Mail, magazines and papers were stacked up everywhere, amidst the boxes of unpacked goods and signs of every day living. How much of this was a result of dementia and how much was merely a product of lazy male bachelorhood, was hard to say.

Dad could be firm, commanding and quite logical at certain times and on certain topics. He could still discuss politics with conviction and some acumen. He was often sure of what he wanted and whom he wanted to be with. He always knew just what he wanted to eat, and he was unswerving in his devotion to Annie and his desire to marry and be with her, always.

On the other hand, he was vague, at best, and confused at worst, on matters such as finances, family history, legal matters, geography and the status of his own affairs. This was particularly true when he was at his own apartment with us and Annie was not present. Television, long a mainstay of Dad's life, was a good barometer of his situation. He could explain quite thoroughly, the difficulties he had with getting his cable hooked up and arranging just the right package of channels at an acceptable price. He could watch his favorite shows with gusto. Yet, he had not a clue as to how to adjust anything on the television set, and when left alone, could often be found watching without comprehending.

While I was staying at his condo, Dad called me in as I got out of the shower one morning, to join him in watching a very exciting and dramatic movie. As I toweled my hair dry, I realized he had been watching the channel that shows nothing but previews, over and over again. He had apparently been watching it all night.

Peculiar sleeping habits are, apparently, another symptom of the Alzheimer's patient. Dad insisted that Alan and I each take a bedroom, which we objected to, as he only had two. He admitted that, when home, he usually fell asleep on the big couch in his living room, watching the TV for company. This made some sense, except that periodic checks through the night indicated that he was mostly up watching the preview channel, taking only occasional catnaps. Upon consultation with Annie, we found that even at her house, he usually slept in a big chair in the living room.

The clincher was the night I got up at about three in the morning to go to the bathroom Dressed only in my boxers, I decided to sneak a peek at Dad in the living room. As I tiptoed in, he looked up from the couch and smiled, and asked, "Are you going back to Virginia now?"

"Yes, Dad. I figured since it is so warm here that I could head back in my shorts. I'll send for the rest of my things later."

We shared a laugh, but I got the point.

As carefully as I could, I started going through Dad's mail, and, delicately asked if I could see his checkbook. His bills were all getting paid, his cabinets had some food, his car had gas; many things seemed, on the surface to be all right. Of course, Annie had been watching out for many of these things, so it was hard to tell. Dad had a nice balance in his checking account, which was good and bad at the same time. Always an addict for sweepstakes, lotteries and the like, Dad was getting several pieces of mail every day soliciting small fees, magazine subscriptions and various purchases, as gateways to fabulous winnings in a multitude of contest formats. Again, Annie had complained of my father's obsession with these sweepstake games, but he had explained the sweepstakes entries away as a harmless hobby, that cost him little or nothing and kept him busy. While no single expenditure was more than a relatively few dollars, these were adding up. Months later, after lots of investigation, I realized just how bad this had become.

Then there were the charities. Every stack of mail included numerous requests from charities all over the world. Please understand that my father's daily mail delivery probably rivaled that of Michael Jordan. Only Dad wasn't getting fan mail: he was getting those sweepstakes announcements, along with charity solicitations and magazines, stacks of them, on an incredible range of topics. Going to the mailbox and sorting the mail was also the highlight of my father's day. How could I rob him of his magazines and sweepstakes? He promised to stop subscribing to new magazines and entering sweepstakes until we could review his finances more thoroughly on my next visit in a month or two. Beware of the sweepstakes, even those that trumpet, "free entry". Most require a "handling fee" or some other kind of processing payment.

Dad absolutely refused to have anyone take over his finances, or even to go into any depth in explaining how he was spending his money. I was sure that a more thorough search of his apartment would yield at least some useful information, but Dad was not amenable, and did not sleep, so what was I to do?

The car would not be an issue for a while, because it was in the shop, towed there by AAA. I got the name and number from Annie and asked them to fix the car. My father's mechanic informed me that this was not his first fender bender, that he had been coming in with alarming regularity. I asked if he would hold the car until I gave him the word to let Dad have the car again.

"Tell my father you're having trouble getting some parts, if he calls," I said, not realizing how difficult it would be to keep my father from picking up the car on his own and driving it. Eventually, under constant harassment from Dad, which included Dad taking a cab to the shop and trying to leave with the car, the mechanic called me. We decided that he would somehow disable the car, to avoid any unauthorized driving by my father.

As we prepared to leave Florida, I was sure of several things.

We would keep the car away from Dad; I would call on a daily basis; I would contact the bank to try and get a better handle on his finances; and Annie, God bless her, agreed to have him stay with her, until I could figure out a more permanent solution. My brother and I agreed that we would need to take an active role in getting Dad's situation worked out, at least enough to protect his health and finances.

I knew I needed help, on the health, legal and financial fronts. It would have to be help that both Dad and I trusted, which might be the best trick of all. I wondered if there was anyone that Dad would trust, and doubted that we would find someone who appealed to both of us.

Once upon a time, we had agreed about most everything, most especially the virtues of our beloved New York Yankees.

Chapter Three

Did I Forget Something?

Yankee Stadium, The Bronx, New York, October 1958: What Do You Think of Bauer, Now?

I close my eyes for just a moment and it is 1958. I am looking up at the large man sitting next to me and we are sharing a laugh like two grownups. The man is wearing a faded blue New York Yankees baseball cap and his eyes are twinkling. The noise of the crowd is almost overwhelming, but I can still hear the man's laughter, as we share this special moment. This is the first World Series game for either of us...also the first adult laugh we have shared together. I am having the best time of my life, which thus far has been all of eight years.

My father and I made many trips together to see baseball games at Yankee stadium, and I remember most of them, as they were all special. But this game, the third game of the 1958 World Series, was the most special of all; I can see, hear and taste almost every minute of that game. The Series was a rematch of the 1957 championships between these same two teams, the Yankees and the Milwaukee (now Atlanta) Braves. The Braves had broken many a New Yorker's heart by winning the 1957 Series, and had bolted to a fast start in 1958 by winning the first two games in Milwaukee. There would be no shame in losing to this team, the Braves of Hank Aaron and Warren Spahn and Lew Burdette and Eddie Matthews. But we really did not want to lose two years in a row, especially since most loyal Yankees fans expected nothing less than a World Series win every year, especially those of us who were eight years old.

The sun had never shown so bright and the grass on the field, always natural in those days, had never been so green. Don Larsen, a good but not great pitcher - despite the perfect game he had thrown in the World Series two years earlier - was on the mound for the Yanks. His job was to keep them out of a devastating three games to none hole. Little did I know that someday I would have a wife who loved to laugh at the statistics that tell you how impossible it would be to come back from a three games to none deficit. I did know that "we" could not afford to lose this game.

Of course I had been in a state of euphoria all day, and would have been, win or lose. Our income did not normally support attendance at sold-out championship series, but a client of my father's had given us the tickets as a present. Good seats, too, just behind third base. That game, that sunny day, the hot dogs I ate, the game program, the cap and ball that my father bought me...they all contributed to the greatest high one can experience: one of pure joy.

And the moment I was remembering, the shared laugh, was one of the best things about that day. You see, a man a few rows down from us had been riding the Yankees veteran right fielder, Hank Bauer, all day. I think Bauer had misjudged a fly ball early in the game, and the guy near us had been merciless in his needling. He called Bauer a bum and far worse, every time he came to bat or fielded a ball. The man was a lout, and a fair weather fan, and his carping at Hank Bauer had worn thin on everyone. Late in a close game, Hank Bauer hit the home run that put the Yankees ahead to stay. As Bauer rounded third base, showing his finest home run trot, another man near us, who had been very quiet up to that point turned toward the loudmouth Bauer critic and yelled in his best New York voice, "So, wuddya think of Bauer now...you asshole?"

I laughed before I could think about it. Then I looked at my dad, and realized that maybe I should not have been laughing at such profanity. Just ignore the comment, I thought. Our eyes met, and I saw that Dad thought the incident was funny too. And we both burst out laughing, two grownups sharing a ridiculous moment in sports that was too funny to ignore. Neither of us said a thing; we didn't have to. I could see his face, round with laughter, as if it were yesterday. My father was not a chuckler; when he laughed, which he did often, he so in robust fashion. The Yankees cap he wore shook and bounced a little on his head when he laughed that day. I was afraid the cap would fall off; my father did not wear caps much, and maybe this was why. The cap stayed on, and the moment moved on to become a savored memory; and the Yankees won that World Series in seven games.

Fairfax County, Virginia, October 1996: Yankees and Braves, redux

The moment I was experiencing in the present, almost forty years later, also passed. I opened my eyes and saw a man in a faded Yankees cap laughing. This man too was my father. Only we were sitting in his dormitory style room in the nursing home, he was wan and pale, and he was laughing at a margarine commercial. Worst of all, I could see his eyes this day too, and those eyes that had twinkled so in 1958 were now dead - there was nothing behind them. They were no longer windows to a man's mind; they were simply organs of the body responsible for sight.

We had been watching the World Series together on television, and it was the Yankees and Braves, now of Atlanta, which may have been what sparked the memory. But the game itself seemed a mystery to my father. The commercials, with their noise and silliness got his attention. Sitting here with Dad was kind of like watching the game with a really little kid. He even had some of his dinner stuck to his shirt, much like a toddler might. This was one of those moments with Alzheimer's that was almost too much to bear.

I had relished the opportunity to watch a ballgame on TV with Dad, thinking that the World Series was something we could still enjoy together. I always seized on anything that appeared to hold Dad's interest, and constantly looked for activities that Dad was able to manage. I've heard other children of Alzheimer's patients say that they hate to give up on having a relationship with their declining parent, and I agree. You can still find ways to enjoy your time together, and, with hard work, you can find things to do together that still bring both of you pleasure. Generally, these activities must be fairly simple, and have the best chance of success if they hark back to a familiar past. Watching baseball on television appealed to me as meeting those requirements. It worked, after a fashion.

We were able to sit in fairly comfortable companionship, watching the game, me never sure how much Dad really did comprehend. We even talked a bit about the game. Yet somehow I could not escape the realities of our situation. Dad did not want to watch the game in the community room, so we stayed in his room. The sterility of that room kept you grounded, and the periodic noise of residents passing by and babbling, never let you forget where you were. The bed I sat on was hard, but perfectly made up, like any good hospital bed. The sink in the corner was an inescapable token of the context for our evening.

Strangely enough, it was another patient who confirmed for me the evocative power of sports memories. There was an older man at my father's nursing home who always hovered about when we visited, but would never speak, or in any way acknowledge our presence. He always seemed on the verge of saying something, but resisted every enticement we could thing of to converse. I was briefing Dad on one of the games that was on television a few nights earlier, hoping for some sign of recognition. I was always looking for familiar things that might help pass the time and maybe spark a little bit of that light that had gone from his eyes.

Smack in the middle of my narrative, which the other man had followed intently, the man broke in with, "Yeah, Cox (the Braves manager) never should have taken Neagle (the Braves pitcher) out so early." He went on to say, in a rush of chattiness, "That damned relief pitcher killed them!" He clearly had known exactly what had gone on during the game...but none of my entreaties could pry one more word from him. I never heard the man say another word.

While wrestling with the relatively mundane question of how to discreetly clean the food off my father's shirt, I realized that I needed to find a better way to protect his shirt and pants from the constant assaults by stray food items that left him looking like the loser in a fierce food fight. In the process of working through this issue, the larger question that had bugged me for two years resurfaced: how do we take on the role of protector for a parent who is suddenly as helpless as a baby? The overwhelming stress of the past two years had increasingly been the challenge of insuring the physical safety, as well as the financial and emotional well being, of the man who had made me feel safe for all of my childhood and for most of my adult life.

Could I ever feel that I had protected my father, the way he made me feel safe and protected on that sacred day at Yankee Stadium and so many times before and since?

That question had haunted me for roughly two years...especially in the early days of realization, as my world came crashing down and I realized that my father could no more function totally on his own than could my two young children. I had started coping with this challenge in earnest before I even left Florida in January of 1995, and knew I had decisions to make as soon as I got home after that fateful trip to see Dad. Once again, my mind drifted back, only this time to a more recent memory, that of just under two years ago, when all the tough decisions started.

There had been so much to cope with, that it was overwhelming, even paralyzing. Where would Dad live, how would he get around? How would he eat, shop, dress? Was there anything that could be done, medically? Where did my father stand financially, and how could I find out? How much did I need to take over my father's life, and how much could he be allowed to remain independent? Why wasn't there anyplace I could go for these answers?

First of all, I needed to prioritize and organize, if I was to have any chance of dealing with this in a remotely satisfactory manner. Knowing this helped some, because the simple act of getting organized was, in itself, somewhat reassuring. I knew that the issues of health and living arrangements were paramount. I had to know just what the medical community could tell me about Dad's condition and what our options were, if any, for getting some kind of medication or treatment. Almost at the same time, I would have to find an alternative living arrangement, as I could not leave Dad totally on his own, and parking him at Annie's was neither satisfactory, nor fair to Annie.

In all, we got the opinions of three sets of doctors. I contacted Dad's long time family physician, who had been seeing Dad regularly for at least ten years, and who had seen him recently for his sore throats and such. He sounded stricken, but admitted that he was finally forced to downgrade his long-term prognosis. He semi apologized for laying my father's symptoms off on mental anguish, but insisted that this had been a reasonable diagnosis for some time. Unfortunately, he was forced to agree that the accumulating evidenced pointed to a degenerative condition and worsening dementia. The dementia was almost certainly caused by Alzheimer's. He would start Dad on the most commonly prescribed drug for that period, in the hopes that it would slow down the progress of the disease and its symptoms.

This was one of the frustrations I encountered with modern medicine. Both the diagnosis and treatment of Alzheimer's are iffy, at best. As noted earlier, the only sure way to know if a patient has Alzheimer's has been post mortem (after death) as the dementia alone is not proof positive. Doctors rely primarily on the symptoms they can observe, and, more importantly, on the anecdotal evidence presented by family and friends of the patient. As the disease wears on, there are certain characteristics that are fairly typical of Alzheimer's, and these can help confirm the initial diagnosis. One such Alzheimer's trait is apparently the manner in which the patient deteriorates.

Alzheimer's patients tend to worsen from plateau to plateau, sinking dramatically, finding a level, and maintaining that level for a while, before sinking dramatically yet again. This contrasts with other aging diseases, which more typically see the patient lose memory and cognition in a gradual, evaporative type process. Incidentally, there are no defined or even typical lengths to these stages, as they seem to vary from patient to patient. The doctors do seem to have names for the stages, level one, level two, etc. There are little more than theories as to what triggers the descent from one stage to a lower one, and I now have my own to add to those of the doctors and researchers.

I firmly believe that change helps trigger the onset of new, lower stages of awareness and independence. This is especially true as familiar surroundings, routines and people are removed from the patient. Every time we moved my father, he suffered an almost immediate, and invariably dramatic, change for the worse. Generally change affects the older population adversely, and, generally, there is some period of adjustment. Even with the Alzheimer's patient, there is supposed to be a rebound effect after a period of adjustment to the new surroundings. But, in my father's case, the rebounds were never enough to get him back anywhere near to where he was before the move.

Thus, you are always balancing the need for progressively more intense care, with the knowledge that the move itself will somewhat degrade your parent's condition. But more on this later.

Back to the health issue, for the moment. We had sought the opinion of a specialist who had worked on my father when he had prostate problems several years earlier. While this was not a case for an urologist, he did see a lot of older patients and had a history with Dad. He felt that he change in my father's mental condition was alarming, and required attention. While reluctant to put a name to the problem, he felt strongly that we should see a neurologist and recommended one.

Annie took Dad to the neurologist, and I conferred with the physicians who had treated Dad during his brief stay at the hospital. The hospital had, in fact, ordered psychiatric evaluation for my father, so concerned were they about his lack of cognitive abilities. Both the neurologist and the hospital told me that they must assuredly conclude that Dad's dementia certainly resembled the symptoms of Alzheimer's. They asked if I was interested in any of the experimental drugs on the market, to which I replied, sure...give me a call with the details.

The drug of choice in 1995, could only, at best, retard the advance of the disease. It could do nothing to reverse the symptoms or to cure Alzheimer's. The popular drug treatment could only delay the inevitable. There were some experimental treatment programs that I would soon learn more about. This ties in with the decisions about living arrangements, as the decisions have significant impact, one upon the other.

You cannot enroll a patient in most experimental drug treatment programs for Alzheimer's if he is living in an unsupervised environment. The patient, in fact, must have 24 hour a day supervision, due to the risk of side effects with most experimental drugs. The programs I was briefed on all had warnings about the dangers of digestive or excretory system failures, which were considered unlikely, but not totally implausible. I spoke with the hospital about the programs they were running and was also contacted by a clinic that was testing some new Alzheimer's drugs, referred to me, I think, by either the hospital or my Dad's doctor.

The intriguing aspect of the experimental drugs was that they were expected to help slightly reverse, not just inhibit the development of the dementia caused by Alzheimer's. This held out some hope of making gains, even if they were marginal, against the loss of memory and awareness, rather than just slowing the loss of same. Though not touted as anything resembling a cure, the newer drugs did hold out hope of moving forward, as opposed to just slowing Dad's backward slide. Given that the rate of movement for this disease is not fixed, such treatment raised my expectations that maybe, just maybe, we could keep Dad in fairly good shape for at least several years. Decisions had to be made quickly, because the key to achieving any noticeable success with most of the aggressive drug treatments is catching the disease early. The giant catch was the need for 24-hour supervision. How was I to arrange that, I wondered?

In the absence of a wife, the only options were to institutionalize Dad, or to hire full time help. Even a wife, or girlfriend, was not a preferred option for the drug testers, as they really wanted a trained health care professional supervising the participating patients. There were problems with both options. Though we had no firm handle on his finances, I suspected that Dad could not afford long term full time help...at least not yet. The cost would run something in the neighborhood of $3,000 to $4,000 per month, on top of his mortgage, medication and other living expenses (utilities, food, etc.). I did not want to institutionalize Dad because he was not yet so far gone as to merit this drastic action, and I feared that such an arrangement, in itself, might set him back. This meant that we were faced with a paradox: most aggressive drug treatments required 24 hour supervision, which was prohibitively expensive at home, and we did not want to move Dad to a full time care residential facility for fear of setting him back. Subsequent events proved that fear to be well founded. In the meantime, we had to pass on the experimental drug, and opted for the more conventional treatment.

I felt that Dad was still not a danger to himself, and my daily phone conversations had convinced me that he still enjoyed a reasonably happy life (though this was largely a result of spending time with Annie), so I searched for halfway measures. For the time being, we decided to leave Dad in his apartment and have a caregiver come in during the day. This person would take care of his meals, make sure he took his medications, and could handle some light cleaning.

Chapter Four

By the Beautiful Sea

South China Sea (or somewhere nearby), September 1942: The
Killer Bees

[What follows is a true story, as recounted to me by my father]
The salty water felt colder than he had thought it would, as he
bobbed up and down in the darkness, his mouth tasting more and
more of the sea. He had never been swimming at night, but had
always thought it sounded like a very romantic thing to do...at least
when it was Coney Island where he contemplated the swim. But
now, wearing clothes, and bobbing rather then swimming, he did not
find the ocean at night to be the least bit romantic or exciting.

He bobbed, rather than swam, for he was buoyed in the water by
the army issue life vest, known as a Mae West. Once again, something
that sounded far better in principle than in practice. In fact, no one
had ever seriously expected to don one of these unwieldy
contraptions, but now here he was, suspended with his head just
above the flapping water, with his arms draped over Mae's generous
air pockets. Worst of all, he was not in the water with a voluptuous
actress, nor with his more moderately proportioned girlfriend from
the Bronx, but rather with hundreds of similarly bobbing fellow
soldiers, none of whom were any better prepared for their midnight
swim than he was.

Uppermost in his mind was survival. There had been no training
for what to do after your ship sank, and he felt even less confident
about any available course of action than he had about the many
aspects of life in the Army-Air Corps that had been thrust upon him

49

after enlistment. He had rushed to join the army straight from a long day of classes at rabbinical college, knowing that the Nazis and Japanese had to be stopped, and spurred on by the rumors that Jews were suffering unimaginable horrors in Europe.

He remembered how his father had enlisted in the U.S. Army during World War I, mostly to demonstrate how much he adored his adopted homeland, as opposed to Grandpa's feelings about the Eastern European nation of his birth. He had never regretted his own decision to enlist, though right about now, he was wondering whether it had been particularly well thought out. After all, he much preferred sitting behind his army-issue field radio, guiding in bombing raids, and sometimes even taking hostile fire, rather than taking an unscheduled swim.

He was annoyed to think that most people never realize how unpleasant a swim in your clothes can be, a fact that was exacerbated by the wool army uniform that had gone into the water with him. Now he felt mostly wet, cold, and angry, as he floated, bobbing in the South China Sea, supported by his Mae West, and wondering how long he would have to endure this particular unpleasantness. Realizing that impatience would not be a productive feeling, he allowed himself to find a serene place, where being alive was the main thing he thought about.

While the details were hazy, in the way they can be when you are smack dab in the middle of a catastrophe, he did know for sure that his troop ship had been hit by a Japanese torpedo, fired by a submarine that they never saw. He knew, or at least was pretty certain, that a lot of his shipmates, many of them good buddies, were dead. He knew this because he had watched so many of them leap from the rail of the sinking ship, rather than lowering themselves down, as they had been hastily instructed to do. Fear, though not quite of panic proportions, had gripped the troops being transported, even though many were battle-hardened warriors. None had been prepared for the terror of having their ship blown out from under them on the high seas.

He wasn't sure how many feet it was from the deck of the ship to the water below, but he was certain that it was a long way...longer than a human body in free fall could tolerate, even if its destination was water. He also knew, because all around him were soldiers who were now bodies, rather than people.

For all the terror that should have gripped his gentle soul, he found himself leaning back gently into that calm place that his conscious mind had found. He was alive, of that he was still fairly certain, and as time went by, more and more of his buddies were dog paddling by to say hello, and "...wadduya make of this?" Maybe, just maybe, this would turn out to be an adventure to tell his kids about one day, after all. He actually dozed off, secure in the arms of Mae West.

He awoke to the sounds of bees buzzing all around him...at least that's what it sounded like. His first inclination to was to wave his arms to swat them away, hoping to avoid being stung, and to shut the sound out by driving the bees away. Unhappily, he began to realize by the light of the rising sun, that many of his comrades were being stung by the bees, as bright red patches appeared on faces where the stings were hitting, and heads began to loll forward, backward and to the side, unnaturally. The bees were rounds being fired by Japanese planes, planes who had been called in by the submarine to finish off the survivors of the sinking troop ship.

One by one soldiers around him succumbed to the bees, and still he bobbed on in the water, helpless to flee or assist his comrades. He thought that he should now, truly be afraid, but it was not fear that filled his mind now, but anger. "Bastards!" he thought. After all, the enemy had already sunk their ship and caused most of his shipmates to die? Why did they have to come back and finish off the helpless survivors?

He never even thought about the fact that the bees might sting him, and that he could be their next victim. He would tell the story years later, and deny that this was courage. Rather, he attributed it either to naiveté, or to the mind's own defense system, a system that filled him only with survival instincts. More than once he did the only thing that was open to him: dog paddling into a group of dead

51

soldiers, and staying very still, hoping that the strafers would think him dead, too. After a time, the bees stopped.

When the buzzing melted away, he reverently pushed aside the comrades whose bodies had helped with his camouflage, and looked around to assess the casualties. He was relieved to find that a friend, Morty, like him a Jewish kid from the Bronx, was still alive. Morty paddled over and compared notes on how he felt, wondering why God had decided that the two of them should live, when so many others had died. Morty also pointed out that three of their other buddies from the City - New York, of course - had not been so lucky.

That was all he remembered before finally falling asleep in the warm afternoon sun.

Soon, he was no longer bobbing in the China Sea, but was at the Passover table in his father's house in the Bronx, awaiting the ceremonial dinner known as the Seder. All six of his older brothers were there, as were all of the wives, and several children. His mother, still the guiding matriarch of the family at seventy, was rushing to get the ceremonial dishes on the table before the men grew restless. She had consented, for the first time, to allow the wife of her oldest son, the matriarch in waiting, to assist her, as she was, at last slowing down. His father stood, now slightly bent over, at the head of the table, eager to start the Passover Seder. The Old Man was not in good health, already in the early stages of cancer, but not conceding a thing to the pain, except for his slight stoop.

The Seders were always more special than any other dinner. Even more than usual, a Seder night brought families together, and the atmosphere virtually begged for discussion and debate, two commodities never in short supply in a large Jewish family. This was such a family, and one that spanned a crucial generational divide, being composed as it was of both immigrants and native born Americans. His parents had both come through Ellis Island, though at different times and from different places. The gap between Polish Jews and Russian Jews was never more apparent than in a family like this, with the more patrician ways of the Poles obvious in his mother's demeanor, and the more relaxed ways of the Russians reflected so clearly in his father's easygoing nature. Though the father never faulted the mother, nor ever considered pointing out the glee with which her native land had turned upon the Jews, the mother often chided the father for being too relaxed, and did not hesitate to point out the indignities visited upon the Russian Jews by Czars and Communists alike. It was all right with all of them; it was just her way.

After a short time the taste of white-hot horseradish had burned its way through everyone's sinuses that the heated words had followed. The younger generation, most of them already established in the world of business, argued for a tough American policy toward the Nazis and the Japanese, and favored swift, and total commitment of the American war machine. The elders, already unwilling witnesses to the horrors of war, were not so quick to support another world conflagration. He was the very youngest, the only one still in school, and he had his own point of view.

To the consternation of everyone else at the dinner table, he proclaimed his intention to enlist in the U. S. Army, become a pilot, bomb the enemy into submission, and then either return to make his fortune in New York, or possibly emigrate to a restored Jewish homeland, if one could be established. If need be, he would fight again, after the Germans were defeated, and go to help found a new Israel, evicting the British and anyone else necessary to free Palestine and create a Jewish state.

Such bold statements, especially from the youngest at the gathering, were greeted as heresy. After all, the youngest of these seven sons, had been consigned to represent the family in the clergy, and was merely two years shy of being ordained as an orthodox rabbi. Furthermore, many in the family questioned how a Jewish state could be created prior to the appearance of a legitimate messiah, as foretold in the Old Testament. The youngest held his tongue for a time, but as they each bit of the dry matzo crackers that signaled the end of the meal, he defiantly stated that Franklin Delano Roosevelt would lead the world to victory over the Nazis, and that a messiah would appear to help restore a Jewish homeland once the first task was done.

Within a year, his father was dead, and he had dropped out of school to enlist in the Army. Two years after that he was dreaming of a family meal in the distant past, while bobbing in the cool water of the China Sea.

The buzzing of bees brought him swiftly awake, but in his confusion he wondered why his alarm was going off at night. In a minute he realized that he was far to wet to have been awakened by the noisy, large, round wind up alarm clock near his bed. He rubbed his eyes to banish the sleep from them, and stung them with salt water. Now, he was wide-awake. Above he could not help but see the fireworks, not of Coney Island on the 4th of July, as he had first imagined, but instead the tracer bullets that were buzzing toward him and his bobbing comrades, as the Japanese fighter made another pass. The bullets lit up the sky so beautifully, that it was hard to imagine that they were, in fact, harmful, no...deadly. The cries of wounded American soldiers competed in the night air with the bees, as more of his friends, and soldiers he had never met were struck, one after another. For some reason, maybe the blackness around him, this attack terrified him more than the one that afternoon had. He still did not expect to die, but the thought of all the others who had and would die, helpless, in the water, made his insides grow cold.

The swarm of bees was really close now, as they seemed to collectively concentrate on this section of ocean, and on these few remaining live Americans. As the nimble airplane dove low for a better look, he felt he could see the face of the young pilot as the flyer's eyes scanned the target area. Perhaps it was illuminated under the plane's canopy by a light on his control panel, but whatever happened, the prey got a glimpse of the predator. He was struck by how young the face looked...and by how much he hated the boy it belonged to.

A bee buzzed close, brushed his forehead with its stinger, and all went black. When his eyes next opened, they were not half way around the world from home, but just a few miles from his cousin's house in Brooklyn, swimming off the beach at Coney Island. This was one of the first great urban amusement parks, complete with all the delightfully tawdry fun that the boardwalk could bring. He was always careful to visit Nathan's for a Coney Island hot dog or three, after swimming, and not before, just as his mother had repeatedly cautioned, to avoid stomach cramps in the water.

The day had been glorious, warm and sunny, especially for September, and the girl his cousin had fixed him up with had been remarkably cute, and what's more, seemed to genuinely like him. He was swimming out to a floating pier, showing off his strong arms and shoulders, and feeling like a million bucks. He reached the pier in a surprisingly short time, and hoisted himself up, expecting to come face to lovely face with Sarah Rosenfeld, but was about to get the shock of his life. Waiting for him on the slippery boards of the pier was the long, pointed face of Rabbi Hirsch, one of the headmasters at school.

Rabbi Hirsch had waited for him to get himself completely up on the pier before he said,

"Good day to you, Shlomo, how are you? You certainly are a strong and graceful swimmer...a talent I never imagined you possessed. It is certainly my good fortune to run into you on this beautiful afternoon, here at the beach. How lucky of you to be able to enjoy this nice warm water, and the company of your friends, instead of being cooped up in that stuffy old school with a bunch of sweaty, rabbis. That's all right, close your gaping mouth, you don't need to say anything...just enjoy the day. Oh, and by the way, you are expelled, permanently from the Yeshiva."

He had invested fourteen grueling years in this pursuit, now over.

In shock, the banned student had fallen from the small floating pier back into the water. His parents would die...no, actually, it was he who was most likely to die, once his mother found out. He bobbed, helplessly, in the water, fighting off the chill and the tendency for his soaking wet clothes to pull him down. But of course, he was not at Coney Island in the past, but fighting for his life in the China Sea, swatting at bees that were really bullets.

By morning the bees had gone, and, somehow, once again, he

had not been stung. The only joy he felt, even at this time of relatively good fortune, was upon discovering that Morty too, lived on. They talked, talked for hours, hoping to forget about their plight, needing to keep their minds off the possible return of the bees, while they waited for rescue.

By the fading light of the late afternoon sun, both soldiers fell asleep. He awoke in the bathtub, with the sound of his father's huge radio filling his ears, describing the exploits of space hero Flash Gordon in the living room nearby. Never one to miss Flash, he hurried through his bath, dried quickly, and shrugged into his pajamas to run into the living room, where the radio stood as a king, towering above all else in the room.

As he ran, still dripping, through the doorway to the living room, he was shocked to see the form of a strange man bending over the radio. Even from behind, he could tell that this was not his father or any of his brothers; it was a stranger. As the stranger lifted himself up from the radio, and slowly turned to face him, he got a greater shock than he had that day at Coney Island. The face of the man was that of the pilot who had tried to kill him in the China Sea.

Hatred so foul that it almost took his breath away, roiled up in him as he strode forward to meet the pilot. He stood there for a full minute, staring into the empty eyes of his adversary, knowing that in a moment he would have the chance to gain revenge, not for himself, but for all of the comrades that had died in the sea.

His hands curled gradually into fists, close by his sides, and he unconsciously moved forward onto the balls of his feet. Now they stood, just inches apart, eye to eye, nose to nose. He could see the shiny black hair on the pilot's head, and it was wet like his. The thought of any similarity between them brought his boiling anger to the point of losing control.

"I'll kill you, you sonovabitch..." he said, as his fists came up and battered the pilot in the stomach and chest. The face would come next, especially as the pilot was bending over from the pummeling, trying vainly to move away and shield himself from the attack.

Suddenly, there were a dozen arms around him, restraining and comforting him at once. He was pulled away from the pilot, whose face had changed dramatically. The face was no longer that of a young Japanese pilot, but that of a badly wrinkled old man, with little hair, no energy, and almost no will to fight back... Shouting people seemed to be coming from everywhere, some sounding angry, others frightened. His robe had come open, revealing his shorty pajamas. He was being led off toward a large sofa, where he was half pushed, and half guided to a seat.

Sitting next to him, and holding his shoulder, no, hugging him was a man he recognized, or thought he did. It was his father, no, not his father...his own son – me - nearing fifty myself.

"What happened, Dad? Were you back in the war again? It's all right now, you're safe. We're in the nursing home, together, and your grandson is just over here." He knew all this to be true, just as surely as he knew that everything that had happened from Coney Island, to the South China Sea, was true, though those truths lay in a different time and place.

That is what Alzheimer's does: it does not just make you forget, it alters one's perception of time, place and perspective, so that the reality of today intermixes, indiscriminately, with the reality of the past, and with the hallucinations of today, to craft a distorted world that seems as real as the one we once knew when our brains were supposed to be functioning normally.

During this fantastic haze, the haze that had been not murky, but tantalizingly real, that Dad had actually re-lived not one, but three different experiences from the past, almost seamlessly. None of them had been distinguishable from the present. The upshot was that Dad had attacked an old man, who had done little more than stare at him, with no particular malice.

Chapter Five

Tell Me Again, Which One of Us Has Alzheimer's?

This chapter will not start with a flashback, as I have made you wait long enough for the thoughts I have that may help answer some of your questions. We will return to the past in just a little bit, but for now, here are some ideas about your situation. I will start by returning to the first five questions I posed in the first chapter.

Is my father all right/are we doing all we can?

No, your father is not all right. Once you and the doctors conclude, not always at the same time, that the patient has Alzheimer's, you have reached a terrifying conclusion, and one that can have no happy ending. Having said that, there are some mitigating factors. There are not, to my knowledge, degrees of Alzheimer's; one does not have a mild or serious case of Alzheimer's. There are, however, stages of this progressive disease.

The inescapable path for the patient is decline over time. Nevertheless, early stages are far less intrusive and disabling than one might think, and if handled right, the patient can still enjoy life and have meaningful interaction with loved ones. The problem lies in the unpredictability of the stages of the disease. Since Alzheimer's generally progresses in jumps, rather than in marginal increments, you may see a big change in your loved one, almost literally in a span of 24 hours, often following a relatively long span of consistent behavior. Adding to your confusion is the fact that the stages have no set or even average duration and often proceed at irregular intervals, meaning that any attempt to predict the patient's decline is pretty much fruitless.

The previous paragraph may sound impersonal and even clinical; unfortunately, that is the way of Alzheimer's. It is an equal opportunity destroyer, striking all kinds of people from all kinds of backgrounds, and yet fickle in the way it moves forward once it takes root. Thus, the doctors could not give me much guidance on how long my father would be self sufficient, nor how long any given plateau was likely to last. At one point, they were surprised at how well he was holding on to a semblance of normalcy, yet six months later they were equally shocked over how much he had degenerated in a two week span of time.

This wreaks havoc with your ability to adjust to your father's behavior, not to mention your ability to provide a safe and secure environment for him. One should be frightened to think that one day he will be going to the mailbox with eager anticipation of the day's arrivals, and a week later he may not even know what a mailbox is. This is an extreme example, but one that is well within the realm of possibility. Early in my father's situation he was still telling me that he would soon be going back to work and had several exciting projects in development. Even at this point, work of any kind, particularly as an inventor, was well beyond my father's reach, but he still thought about it, and recognized that he had been a successful inventor of toys. In fact, he could, and did, regularly rattle off a list of his most successful inventions and told people, often several times exactly what each of his toys was famous for.

For months, my father kept a stack of file folders with pictures of his toy inventions, awards he had received, copies of his Who's Who listings and related honors, rather neatly organized, and ready for showing. When we started looking at assisted care facilities, he refused to go without his files, which he carried in an old, but still beautiful leather briefcase. He understood that the premier assisted care facilities were hard to get into, and was convinced that his chances of being admitted to these exclusive clubs would be enhanced by the presentation of credentials, which he invariably delivered.

Our exploration of assisted care options lasted only a couple of months, but once he moved, he could not have told you how he had come to be an inventor, what he had invented, or, perhaps even what an inventor was. He had moments of relative clarity, but his overall grasp of who he was declined badly.

My point is this: early on you should not write your parent off, they can still interact and enjoy life, but you must treat him like an alcoholic, who has a chronic condition, which will never really go completely away, no matter how good things may seem at the moment. You are constantly trying to live for the moment, while preparing for the tough road ahead.

This approach applies to all of the health and lifestyle decisions you will have to make for your father, or with him, if he is able. Above all else, you must constantly monitor your father's condition, alertness, awareness and spirits. His ability to harm himself and/or others will be in your hands, and could become an issue very suddenly. This is tough to do, when we don't live close by, which, in turn, affects your thinking about his living situation.

Safety and Sanity (or, Baby You Can't Drive My Car)

How do you know when your father has become a danger to himself and others? This is, of course, a very subjective question, and one not easily answered. What may appear to be a fairly innocuous loss of recent memory, can turn into a deadly characteristic if it manifests itself behind the wheel of a car. As my brother and I found out, even though Dad could still work the controls of his car, and drove for some distances without mishap, his temporary lapses of focus were killing his sense of geography and lane integrity.

Our lives would never be the same. Dad might, from time to time, be fine for routine driving, but could not be trusted unsupervised on an ongoing basis. The fact that putting him behind the wheel endangered others as well as himself, made this a crucial decision about Dad that had to be made, and soon. We vowed never to put him in a position where his confusion would put him in the car headed the wrong way on a road, bearing down on some innocent driver, head on. So, as mentioned earlier, we took the car in to be fixed after his minor accident, and arranged for it not to be returned.

This was to be a bitter and prolonged battle. Dad had been driving for fifty years; he had a spotless driving record, with no accidents and few tickets on his resume; and he lived in a community in Florida where his independence was completely derived from his mobility via auto. We soon found out that Dad's fierce attachment went well beyond the need to feel mobile and independent, though in itself these were powerful forces. For Dad, the threatened loss of his right to drive was a blow to his ego of massive proportions.

Think about it: while most adults complain about traffic, long drives, rude road hogs and so forth, the fact is that we take driving for granted. As teenagers, we all count the days until we get our drivers licenses, and the first days of driving bring an incomparable sense of freedom and pride to our early years. As a father of teenagers, I can see how much they yearn to drive, how much they think about what they want to drive, and how they suffer the passing days slowly dragging by before they can get out on the road. And, just as surely as driving changed my life at sixteen, it will change theirs, hopefully in a safe and benevolent way. Now imagine telling them to think about giving up that blessing, that badge of adulthood! Every limitation that parents impose to restrict the total independence of driving teens frustrates and angers them.

That is what we do to our parents, essentially becoming villains, rather than heroes, as we strip them of their mobility, their independence and a degree of their pride, by taking away their right to drive. The Alzheimer's patient rarely, if ever, will admit that his ability to drive has been impaired, even in the slightest. Some of that is because they fear losing the right to drive, but, for the most part, the erosion of driving ability has escaped their conscious minds.

Dad and I argued, often bitterly, over the idea of him driving again. Initially, he felt that he was, perhaps, temporarily incapacitated, and expected to resume driving as soon as he was better. But he was still aware enough of the world around him to realize that lots of time was passing and that his car was still, mysteriously, in the shop. I made excuses about the car, and told him that he was still not well enough to drive, anyway. Ultimately, I agreed that, when he was sure he was ready, we would re-evaluate the situation. This bought me some time, but did not solve anything. Nevertheless, telling him he was through as a driver would have been like a death sentence to him, so I stalled - though still with no car that he could get his hands on.

Finally, someone told me about a special program, run by an independent group for the DMV, that would give driving tests to those who had been incapacitated, to see whether they had progressed to the point where they were competent to drive again. Many of their clients were older folks; others had been injured, sick or in some way compromised as potential safe drivers. The program would administer driving tests under highly controlled conditions, with no risk to the driver or the tester. In the rare event that the driver passed with flying colors, they could proceed to take a standard DMV test, or, as in many cases, could just resume operating a car under their already valid drivers license.

Dad was thrilled once we had a date for the test and was confident that he would pass with flying colors, as he liked to say. Of course, he failed miserably, and quickly forgot his promise to abide by the test results. It fascinated me that my father could think about that driving test, rationalize why he failed, come up with explanations (which he stuck to from one conversation to the next over several months time) and argue, often persuasively that he should be allowed to drive...yet, he had, by this time, little command over the intricacies of driving. And his failures behind the wheel were not a result of physical inadequacy, but of mental confusion and inconsistent attention to detail.

For three months we discussed and even quarreled, over the issue of driving. I maintained, unfailingly, that my hands were tied, but that I would work on getting him a re-test, due to the extenuating circumstances he had explained. And this is what he had explained, as closely as I can repeat and paraphrase it. He would always begin by saying that, "the bitch (tester) hated me, right from the moment I got there."

When asked why she would hate him, Dad could come up with no reason. But he maintained that she had intentionally tricked him, set him up, asked the impossible, falsified the test results, etc. His complaints included the purported use of an illegal course on a back lot - he was right that this was not a street test; the use of orange cones that were not firmly placed, but moving in the wind - no basis here; the issuing of instructions in rapid fire, random order, which no one could have kept up with - probably true enough to him; and constant questioning by the tester that threw him off - again, that's how he saw it. He also felt that the controls of the car were in very unusual places and supposed that it was a result of the test utilizing a foreign made vehicle "from Russia" that he - and probably no American - had ever seen or heard of before. His nurse, who had accompanied him on the test, pointed out that the car was an Oldsmobile.

She also reminded him, albeit gently, that he had utterly failed to parallel park the car, even after three tries. To this he replied, "So what, no one in Florida can parallel park, it's all malls with pull in spaces." His explanation for failing to slow down or turn when instructed to do so, was, "It wasn't the right time..."

The driving test, controversial as it was, proved to be a godsend. At last, I had the opportunity to deny him access to a car, without appearing to be the bad guy. Still, to keep some semblance of peace, I promised to work on a re-test, and sited a mandatory waiting period as the reason it was taking so long. Maybe I suspected that the time would come when he no longer cared about driving.

In a way, this becomes a pattern with Alzheimer's. As the responsible party, you take things away from the patient's independence, and take the heat for that, and even for the things you are not responsible for. The arguments can be bitter and you get called all kinds of names, accused of stealing money, and more. Yet, over time, Dad came to care about fewer and fewer things, so the arguments over driving, for example, would stop (money was even worse, but I'll save that for a little bit later) leaving you relieved and disappointed, all at the same time.

Dad hated losing his wheels...but he loved telling the story of the driving test. It was almost as if that test became a symbol of all the things that were being unjustly, and inexplicably taken from him, and he was railing against the collective injustice of it all. He got angry telling the driving test story, but he was lucid, and passionate, two traits that would evaporate all too soon.

Sources of Help (or You Better Find a Friend, Fast!)

The worst part of dealing with a declining parent, especially one who is far away, is not having anyone to answer your questions, to advise you, to assess your father's condition - besides a doctor - and to tell you how to deal with all the choices that must be made. You may in fact, have family close by, but they don't really count for two reasons: they are not qualified to deal with the problems of aging, unless they happen to be healthcare professionals, and they are not objective.

You're talking about placing yourself, and the declining parent in the hands of strangers, perhaps literally, and that requires a great deal of faith. We're talking here about where they live, what kind of care they need, how they are treated medically, what kind of supervision they need, and of course, their financial well being.

In my case, I decided that one of the first things that Dad and I needed was an attorney. His legal and financial affairs were clearly a mess, and he was eager to put them in order so that he, eventually I, could at least pay his bills and see to it that he didn't lose everything to the government. Mind you, he was in no way ready to cede control over his affairs, legal or financial, but he wanted an orderly transition to be arranged, and he wanted me to be comfortable with the way it was set up, so that, being the oldest, I could take over when necessary. That was fine with me, and I was prepared to have Dad make all the decisions at the early stages, when all we had taken hold of was the ban on driving.

I called a friend in state government, who made some inquiries, and replied quickly with the name of a firm that was strong in elder care issues and estate management, and with the name of a partner who was well known to the trusted people my friend had talked to. I called and chatted with the attorney, and my first impression, which proved accurate, was that she was both skilled and caring, so I gave Dad her name and vice versa. Since Dad was already a bit undependable about things, I suggested that the attorney call him if she did not hear from him in a week or so. She did call him, and arranged to come by to meet him at his girlfriend's apartment, where she conferred for hours with both Dad and his friend.

Dad's friend had set up a Living Trust, with the help of her son and his attorney, and was very pleased with the arrangement. She felt that such a Trust secured her finances and allowed her son to assist in their management, while still allowing her as much, or as little, input as she wished. With her influence, Dad was persuaded to go the same route, which I approved of, and the attorney kept me informed of their progress, though all the decisions were really Dad's. The attorney made it possible to arrange the trust and other legal affairs in a manner that insured that Dad made the key decisions at the front end; because she made it her business to do so. She did this by working with him at his or his girlfriend's apartment, never at the office; and by setting whole days aside to work with him, so he never felt rushed or pressured. She even brought people from her office to witness documents, when necessary. We were never charged for travel time, or for the time of the witnesses. In fact, the attorney never charged us for any of the extra effort she made so that this would be easier for Dad. Make no mistake: the bills were substantial, but they could have been much worse. She never even charged me the standard one-hour rate for any phone calls I made when there was just that one burning question to be answered. This is a trait to be sought in your attorney, because otherwise, the bills can be overwhelming, especially if you have an attorney who starts the meter running each time you talk, and charges any partial hour at her full hourly rate.

When the angelic attorney - Did I really say that? Does it qualify as a paradox? - called me to say they were basically done, Dad had a

Living Trust, a new will, a Living Will, a healthcare surrogate designation. She had Dad send me a copy of everything, and made sure it happened while she was with him. I will get into the nature of these instruments later. The point is: thanks to a knowledgeable and caring attorney, Dad got things in order, and did so in a way he was comfortable with. All this was accomplished not long after my brother and I went down to Florida to see for ourselves what was going on, and we both felt better, knowing that he was still strong of will, though fading, and that he at least was getting his house in order. This was accomplished not a moment too soon.

The legal and financial arrangements were made infinitely easier by the fact that, forgetful as he was, and though he could be temporarily confused, Dad was still basically, in his right mind and knew his own will and wishes. The attorney was quite confident that this was the case, but for further assurances also had a psychologist, who was an expert in aging and dementia, and who the firm routinely used for such matters, meet with Dad to render an opinion. She concurred that he knew what he wanted done with his finances, his legal affairs, and his body.

I should point out that I did try to contact my father's previous attorney. This made sense, as he should have had a handle on my Dad's legal, and possibly financial situation, and would be the logical starting point. Though he was not an expert on elder care or estate planning, I had envisioned turning to him for assistance, and adding the legal specialists we needed, as appropriate. Interestingly, he had little interest in working with me. In fact, one by one, I found that my father's entire team of advisers, including his accountant and stockbroker, was surprisingly unhelpful.

What I surmised was that my father, whose mind had been going in and out for some time, had been exasperating the people he worked with on financial and legal matters. It's tough enough for family to understand the inconsistencies, the non-comprehension, the forgetfulness, and the quarrelsome nature of the budding Alzheimer's sufferer. Strangers, even if they are professional friends, find it extremely difficult. I had little desire to apologize for my father's behavior, or to make explanations for him. After all, these people all worked on his behalf, and made money through their dealings with Dad, why should I have to beg their forgiveness and cooperation?

Within two weeks of the amenable and efficient conclusion of the legal arrangements with our new attorney, I had fired all of Dad's advisors and hired new ones who were experienced in dealing with aging clients that had declining faculties. The attorney had pulled the new team together, and she also directed me to a private social service agency that assisted me with care for my Dad. That, then, was the starting point for sorting out the technical side of the nightmare.

For information on what resources might be available to you, here are some of the places that I called: local hospitals; local and state government offices on aging; local nursing homes and assisted care facilities; national groups like the AARP; and, of course, there is always the Internet - you can start with your city or county's web page. You should also enter "Alzheimer's" into your Internet browser's search engine. Several useful sites will come up, including some groups started precisely for the purpose of helping Alzheimer's families to connect.

Note: The need for a private social service agency was caused by the relative lack of public healthcare assistance. There are places where state and local health or social service agencies provide a range of care support for sick or aging citizens. In New York, for example, where my parents started out, it was possible to obtain some limited help with in-home care. Of course you do have to pay for such public services in the form of higher taxes. By fleeing to a notoriously low-tax state, my parents opted to lived in a place where most social and health services needed to be purchased from the private service providers. There are always tradeoffs, and philosophies differ from state to state. This just means that you need to investigate your options in the state in which your parent is domiciled. Furthermore, be aware that moving your parent to another state or locality just because it might offer more public services can backfire. There are likely to be residency requirements for eligibility.

Chapter Six

Which Side Does the Salad Plate Go On?

New York, New York, August 1962: New York, New York…It's a
Toddlin' Town

The lights of the George Washington Bridge twinkled ahead of
us, and just beyond, the radiance of New York City shown in the
early morning darkness. The bridge beckoned us toward Manhattan,
and what had been very sleepy eyes began to widen, as I realized
that Manhattan was now just minutes away. Beside me, ever so tall,
sat my father, his confidence behind the wheel concealing whatever
nervousness he might be feeling about the impending sales call we
were about to make.

Within minutes we had raced over the bridge and were headed
for the West Side Highway that ran the length of Manhattan Island.
I was still groggy, but coming awake fast with anticipation of the
day's events. As I peered over the side window, I could see the huge
rock formation created by glaciers thousands of years ago, known as
the Palisades. I thought I could just make out the details of the famous
Palisades Park, an amusement park with a dramatic view of New
York City, made famous by a sixties rock and roll song; the Wild
Mouse ride at the park was destined to live forever in my memory as
the first place I kissed a girl, several years later.

We had an appointment for nine a.m., sharp, at the downtown
offices of one of the largest toymakers in the world, at which I would
help demonstrate my father's latest invention. He loved bringing me
with him to show a real life child interacting with his toy inventions;
he also, as I always suspected, and would later confirm, enjoyed my

company, and it gave him something to focus on besides his dislike of selling.

My father had always loved the inventing part; his mind was constantly racing with ideas, and his hands always found ways to translate them into working models, no matter how unlikely the idea seemed. But to make a living at this, he had to face the inevitable sales call. I was fortunate enough to be his partner on these sales calls, which I loved, both for the excitement of the trip into Manhattan and for the time with my dad.

Although he shunned getting caught up in a nine to five job, and dreaded the idea of commuting into New York on a daily basis, my father loved the city in the early morning. So, he would set his appointments with the toy companies early, and we would get out of bed in the dark before dawn, leaving Rockland County via the New York State Thruway or the Palisades Parkway, long before the rush hour "racers" had started their engines. That way, we could "sneak" back into the city of our birth under cover of darkness, find an easy place to park, and take in a sumptuous breakfast at one of several Manhattan diners that my father had frequented for most of his adult life. These were the kind of restaurants with plates so full of grease that the mere sight of them would have given my mother a heart attack. At this time of day, the massive street sweeping machines would just be finishing their rounds and traffic would be starting to cover the soon-to-be overheated byways of New York.

We would hurry into the already busy little eateries - true New Yorkers are notoriously early risers - knowing exactly what we wanted. Within minutes a waiter wearing a greasy red apron would be bringing us heaping plates of equally greasy food, with heat rising from the plates like the steam that rose each morning from the grates in the street. This particular morning the waiter, whose name happened to be Red, set down two plates in front of me: French toast and eggs covered one round brown plate, and a pile of crusty hash browns sat atop the other. My dad had the same thing; we always ordered the same thing, one of us waiting for the other to order and the just saying, "ditto" to the waiter. At this particular establishment, the waiter named Red, always seemed to wait on us. He was a friend of my father's from some previous life - a neighbor, I think - but actually knew my Uncle Manny better than he did my Dad. It always puzzled me about his name, since there was not a sign of any hair atop the waiter's head, red or otherwise.

Red set the plates down with care, and bantered a bit with my father, the affection obvious in his voice. Dad was always nice to everyone, though he was not a gregarious man with strangers, only with friends. He laughed, as Red made some comment about a little guy like me never having enough room to finish all this food, something along the lines of "his eyes are always bigger than his stomach". Dad laughed easily, but made eye contact with me and quickly let me know that I should eat only what I wanted, and that it would be fine with him, however much I might leave over. We were a couple of "men" on a business trip, after all.

My dad and I talked through breakfast about the upcoming presentation to the toy company moguls. He wondered aloud whether his working model would hold up, as he had been concerned that it might be too frail for a live demonstration. We had to do this now, since the company had said it was already almost too late to make the Spring toy show that opened the next Christmas season, which was actually a year and a half from now, and Dad really wanted to see this particular invention on store shelves by the Christmas after this one. Thus, we would risk the shaky model, and I would be most careful with it. I was asked my opinion of which feature of the toy we should demonstrate first, and as I responded, my chest filled with the pride of being an "expert" partner, rather than a kid, tagging along. After all, I did know my toys!

We had finished eating by 7:30, and I watched as Dad sipped his coffee and smoked half a cigarette. By now, the little diner was filled past capacity, and I entertained myself by studying the myriad people who squeezed around the tables and relaxed up at the counter. I never minded taking a seat at the counter, as it actually afforded the diner more room, and the swivel chairs were great fun.

Dad glanced at the check, and I could see him calculating the tip in his head, which always amazed me as a kid. He set a fan of bills down over top of the check and said what he always did, "Time to go, kiddo", and we were off. An early morning shower had darkened the sky and the street, but just now it had stopped raining and I was enjoying the chug and scrape of busy shoes moving swiftly over the pavement and the symphony of car and taxi horns that were providing a soundtrack to early morning Manhattan.

We headed, as we always did, for Uncle Manny's liquor store near the Chrysler Building. My Uncle Manny had always owned retail shops, but liquor had been his life - not drinking, but selling. Manny had a head for business, and made a small fortune with his little shop by cultivating a steady clientele of business executives who catered their office events with Manny's liquor, and used the finest bottles of Scotch and so forth from Manny's stock as Christmas presents and for other business gifts. Any one firm might order dozens of cases of fine liquor at retail every Christmas and in the Summer, and the executives would do their personal shopping at Manny's too. With his quick wit, and wonderful sense of humor, Manny became fast friends with many of his bigger clients, who often would tip him off to business ventures that seemed too good to be true, yet were honest, and, invariably, right on target.

Manny was a legend in the family for supposedly having made a fortune in his business and in the stock market…and for losing almost as much as he made. As shrewd as Manny was in retail, he was incredibly unlucky, or inept at playing the market. It mattered not one bit to me, for I loved Manny for his funny ways, and clever little gifts. He always called me "Uncle Picklepuss", and greeted me like a long lost son. Manny and his wife had no children of their own, so they "adopted" their many nieces and nephews, and were extraordinarily generous with all of us. Of course, I was his favorite.

We reached the locked front door of Manny's Liquors before eight, and Dad knocked what he called the secret knock. A painfully thin, balding man, wearing a tan merchant's jacket and with a cigarette dangling from his mouth came to let us in. He and Manny were in the back, checking stock (and playing gin), so Jack showed us to the back room. Jack had worked for Manny for years; he loved my uncle and my dad, and Manny trusted him with his store, the only person, other than my aunt, who Manny would leave alone in the store for more than an hour.

The greeting that Jack and my uncle gave Dad, was so genuinely warm, that it made me all the prouder to be with him. They both hoisted me up, making no effort to mask their fondness for me, but it was my dad who drew most of their attention. They wanted a complete briefing on today's presentation, what the new toy did, how it worked, and where the idea had come from. Then Dad had to give them the rundown on the company executives we would be meeting with, and the economic status of the world's largest toy company. And Manny asked the inevitable question about why Dad didn't just give in and accept one of the repeated offers he got to take a job as VP in charge of development for one of these firms, to which he replied, as always, that he was having too much fun.

The presentation merely completed a perfect morning. On this particular day, my father and I were demonstrating an invention that pitted two players against each other in a game that allowed them to match wits in a game of strategy. The theme happened to be one of war battles, which was somewhat inspired by the traditional game of "Battleship". The difference was that this game involved more than simply guessing where the other person's ships were: you had to choose an attack strategy, complete with composition of attack force, route of attack, strategic objectives, etc. The match between your attack strategy and the attack/defense strategy employed by your opponent determined the outcome of each battle. The key to the game was that the matching was conducted electronically and the "computer" determined the outcome.

This might not seem remarkable by today's standards, but remember that this was 1962, that there were no home computers, nor any home video games, at that time. My father, at the top of his game at forty, had "invented" what he referred to as an "analog computer" using metallic grids made out of aluminum foil with holes cut out in strategic places. This system would be engaged by my

Dad ten years later to power the classic home game known as "Monday Night Football", which was named for and endorsed by the pioneering show on ABC. In effect, this became the forerunner of today's football video games, which are among the most popular and exciting products of the home video revolution. Today's kids - and adults like me - have become accustomed to playing football at home, in a game that hinges upon the selections of offensive and defensive plays and the way in which they match up.

The toy company executives called my father's latest invention "brilliant". I had no reason to doubt them.

Throughout the morning drive, the hearty breakfast, the repartee with Manny and Jack, and right on through the make or break presentation to the officers of the toy company, Dad was in total control. Despite his claim of nerves, my dad was on top of the meeting from start to finish, anticipating every question or concern. The sale was made the moment the model of the toy sprung to life in my hands. Dad was all smiles as we left, and he bought us each a giant pretzel from the first street vendor we came to. He always did after one of these presentations, win or lose.

In our joy and general bonhomie, we talked and laughed the entire hour it took to get home. We stopped at the electronics store on the way, to be sure my father had some little gizmos he needed for the new model he was working on, and he added a funny hand-held electric fan for me.

It was early afternoon by the time we got home, and the house already smelled of turkey roasting and numerous side dishes cooking on top of the stove and in the oven. I had almost forgotten that we were celebrating my grandparents' anniversary that night and that my mother's whole family was coming to dinner. As I moved slowly through the intersection of aromas in the large kitchen, I was once again amazed at the total competence of the grownups that oversaw my life. From Dad's mastery of New York and the toy world, I had now transported to my mother's incredible gift for entertaining. Here she was with twelve people expected for dinner, numerous wonderful things in various stages of cooking or baking around the kitchen, a table to set, and a house to prepare, and she was laughing and joking on the phone with one of the neighbors. She had even found time to insure that my brother, Alan, then a tyke of five, had been bathed, scrubbed and hair-gelled into respectability.

When I wandered into the dining room, my amazement grew. The table was already set for twelve with my mom's best china and silver, and the light from the chandelier reflected brightly on the crystal and utensils. Every setting was perfect. But here, my mother showed her one weakness: she never could remember on which side of a place setting to put the salad plate. As always, she asked my father if he remembered, and as usual he responded that he could not see how it would matter. They were so happy that day, over the successful toy sale and the upcoming dinner with family that they both laughed off the challenge of the salad plates. So, there it was: my parents were in complete control of everything, except for the salad plates.

Fairfax County, Virginia August 1996

I walked carefully with Dad toward the dining room, telling him eagerly about the big dinner tonight. It was rare for him to venture all the way downstairs to the dining room, as he usually ate in his room. He was a bit unsteady on his feet, and generally had problems in the big, busy atmosphere of the main dining room. As I gently held his arm in mine to guide him, Dad was telling me how this restaurant we were going to had been a favorite of his and my mother's for many years. He said they had been coming here since before I was born. He wondered aloud why she was not here yet. For a moment he was sure that my son, David, then twelve, was my brother Alan. I was glad, as always, for David's company, and for his patience with the residents who wanted him to be their grandchild.

We found an empty table and a rather large woman, dressed in white, and with a bouffant of flaming hair approached the table. My father's eyes lit up for just a moment, as he greeted her with a weak wave, and a more enthusiastic, "Hey, Red...how ya' doin'?" For just that moment, my father had a bit of the old glow, and he looked at me with something that appeared to be recognition. He did seem to know who I was, which was not always the case these days. But then he asked me why I had not yet hugged my mother, faltering a bit when I hesitated in my reply.

Before I could say anything, he admitted that the woman probably was not my mother, ands asked again, when she would be here. "Red", patted my father on the back rather gently, placed a small glass of grape juice in front of him, and told him to go easy on the "wine" before dinner. Just as my father was asking with growing concern where my mother was, my son approached with bad news. He informed me that the main course for the big dinner that evening was going to be ham, which my father's Kosher upbringing had never allowed him to eat. We realized that Dad would probably not even know the meat was ham, but were trying to respect his lifelong beliefs, and trying to take no chances, since his taste buds might not be afflicted with Alzheimer's.

It was David who saved the day, as he had instructed the staff to substitute the fish sticks for Dad's ham. I thanked goodness for my own kids, who not only helped by virtue of their existence, but who had been wonderful about keeping me company and visiting their grandfather, every week, without being begged or cajoled.

There was a festive air in the dining room, as residents continued arriving and talked, excitedly amongst themselves. The atmosphere was contagious, and it was good to see so many of the other patients busy with anticipation, rather than desperation. Soon, food was arriving, and the relatively good food was generating the kinds of pleasant aromas that might add to the appeal of a pretty decent restaurant.

Just as the food arrived, so did Susan and Diana, and I was so glad to have my wife and daughter join us. I wondered whether Dad would have a clue as to who they were, but knew that either way, they would help get him engaged in conversation. Susan always worked hard at getting my Dad to talk about something, and Diana, at ten, was already quite a conversationalist, able to initiate dialogue in any situation. Dad loved the added attention, especially from these lovely and engaging ladies. He did not seem sure who exactly they were, but took obvious pride in establishing that they were clearly part of his family.

Dad's attention span, however, was short, and soon I noticed that Dad was engaged in conversation with his grandson, trying apparently to figure out exactly who he was, even though David had been there for some time and had already been talking to Dad. At the same time, Dad began playing absently with his fork and spoon. He seemed to grasp who his grandson was, but was having less luck with the eating utensils. He asked me why these "tools" had been left on his "desk", and whether he was going to have to repair that "damned radio" again today. His grandson assured him that the radio was working fine, and demonstrated the proper use of the tools in question.

At the next table, a woman who looked rather young and pretty to be in a nursing home was also struggling with her utensils. She was picking them up, waving them in the air and calling for help. Other residents rushed to her aid, as did two attendants. She was complaining loudly that "they had given her the wrong silver, again" and told them that she could not eat with "stolen" silver, no matter how pretty it was. She was insisting that the police be called in, and when none appeared, she began to toss forks and spoons onto the floor. This, she proclaimed, was where the "counterfeit silver" belonged. It was turning into quite a scene.

My father, who had been watching the growing storm quietly, suddenly spoke up. "Ah, there's your mother, now," and he was pointing at the obstreperous woman with the silverware problem. Just then, Red interceded to help ease the woman into her chair and calm her with a few comforting words. As the poor woman reluctantly acquiesced, Red caught my eye and leaned carefully back toward me.

"What's so sad," she confided, "was that Mrs. Clancy was

once the most celebrated hostess in Northern Virginia. Her dinner parties for a hundred were legendary, and were THE place to be. She was a queen…of sorts…now she doesn't even know how to handle her dinnerware, poor dear."

"Serves her right," snapped my father, for no particular reason.

I could not help but think about how far we had come in this latest downhill spiral.

We had come to the conclusion that Dad needed to be in a full service nursing home, when he had become a danger to himself and, potentially to others. Overcoming my reluctance to remove him from familiar surroundings, I had initially tried assisted care living, which works for many, but was not adequate for Dad. Whether he could have made it there for a while or not, had been rendered moot by the setback he suffered once he moved there. He loved the new place by the sea, but was no longer capable of even basic maintenance functions, once he got there. A good candidate for assisted care the day he moved, progression to the next lower stage of dementia had rendered him almost helpless, which is too far gone for assisted care. This really signaled the end of Dad's days in Florida, where he had fled from New York long ago, and had begged to stay.

Unable to afford, both assisted care AND full time private nurses, we had decided to move Dad, one final time, to a nursing home. This time, we felt that he needed to be nearby, so that Dad and his surroundings could be monitored on a regular basis. I felt the need to personally investigate the home that would undoubtedly become Dad's last place of residence, and wanted him nearby, where my brother and I and our families could spend time with him. I hoped that the advantages of family visits would overcome the drawback of moving one more time to unfamiliar surroundings.

We had flirted, briefly, with the idea of one of us taking him into our homes. The doctors and elder care experts we consulted with had said this was impossible.

Chapter Seven

My House, Your House

Rockland County, New York, December 1960: A-Hunting We Will
Go

My parents stood, silhouetted in the bright screen of sunshine
that lit up the large picture window in the empty living room. I had
to squint to see them as more than dark outlines against the blinding
light, simultaneously noticing the strong smell of sawdust that filled
the air of the still unfinished home. At that moment I realized that
our year of driving to strange locations to see work-in-progress homes
was almost over. The housing development here in Monsey, New
York would be our new home in the very near future.

I was delighted and disappointed, all at the same time. After all,
I had come to enjoy our weekly adventures that took us to remote
sections of Long Island, and northern locations such as Westchester
and Rockland Counties, even so far away as southern Connecticut.
On the other hand, the prospect of actually buying a home and moving
to the undulating lawns and quiet streets of the suburbs held the
promise of freeing me from the concrete ball fields and uncertain
streets of New York City.

I decided to take another look at the downstairs, where I could
greedily survey the large "rec room" that would soon become my
sanctuary. The house was something they called a "split level",
meaning that it was two floors, one partially below ground and one
fully above. One entered at the mid level, with short stairs leading

up to the right and down to the left. Directly above lay the kitchen, dining room and living room, with four bedrooms (quadruple the number of our apartment in the Bronx) down a long hallway to the left. Downstairs lay a huge rec room and a short hallway that led to the two car garage. Through the rec room and out the sliding glass doors lay a modest but adequate back yard that was bordered by a small, man-made lake.

In the rec room, I smiled to myself as I pictured where a pool table would sit, and fantasized about a monster stereo system that would shake the entire house at full volume. I had hauled my three-year-old brother, Alan, downstairs with me so that my folks could conduct serious negotiations with the portly man who was showing us the house. This was always a major step: progressing from the first look at a comfortably furnished model home, to roughing it in a half completed real home, with sawdust on the floors and see-through walls made up only of studs. Of course the next step, if the home passed this test, was to go back to the construction office or model home, to peruse the map of the entire development, in order to see what our real life lot choices might be within the housing development.

My father always tended to be a bit over-anxious, seeing the positive in every home, reflecting his eager desire to get out of the city and make a new life in the suburbs, or the "country" as he tended to call it. My mother was just the opposite, reserving even the most preliminary judgments until she could think through all of the pros and cons. Sometimes I thought that, if left entirely to my mother, we would never buy a house, and if left entirely to my dad, we would have bought the first house we looked at, almost a year ago.

Buying a house would accomplish our ultimate goal, that of getting us out of the city, which was no small thing. I certainly had a good life in New York City, but I yearned for a move that would give me the safety and comfort of green grass to play baseball and touch football, a place where I could swing lazily in a hammock reading a book, or munch on a snack while listening to the competing sounds of the Yankees game on the radio and the buzzing of the insects of spring. My head danced with visions of backyard barbecues and school bus rides with pals, instead of city bus rides with weirdoes.

On the other hand, house hunting, as my parents loved to call it, had become a way of life for the past year. We'd wake up early every Saturday and Sunday morning, race each other to the newspaper, and tear into the real estate section to scan the prospects for the day's itinerary. My father would generally be in charge of reading off the possibilities, while my mother sat at the dining room table with a pad and pencil, writing names of housing developments and directions. Later, she would fill in a collective list of pros and cons for each.

By nine or so each weekend morning we would have our list and by ten we'd be on the road to the first place on the list. We knew that we would soon be meeting all kinds of colorful people and touring the best model homes that each place had to offer. Sometimes we would huddle in a quiet spot outside to review family reactions to the latest model home. I always got a kick out of the furnishings in the model homes, at times wishing that we could just have the model, as is. Of course nearly as many sets of furnishings made us ill and left us wondering whether the decorator was vision-impaired. I remember that one such monstrosity grossed us out with deep purple walls and furniture that looked as though it had been reclaimed from the Salvation Army.

My parents loved the thrill of exploring new places, each little suburban town unfolding before our hungry eyes. Dad would maneuver the Pontiac through the shady streets as we left the interstate farther and farther behind, my mother with map and directions spread out in her lap. Then, and always as if by surprise, we would spy the flags flying over some burgeoning housing development, and would pull up eagerly, at the model home.

I found something to like about every one, probably because nearly all of them beat our cramped apartment in the Bronx and each held the promise of escape from it. Often, it was at least partly my job to keep my younger brother in check, making sure he did not wander off or get into trouble as we toured. My father loved to knock on the walls, giving a knowledgeable nod of his head, as if the knock had yielded vital information about the soundness of the house. This was a trick my mother's father had taught Dad, although the results meant a lot less to my Dad, than they would have to my grandfather.

We looked at some houses on Long Island that were so huge, my mother called them "mansions", and some in Westchester County that had the regal look of "castles". At one model home, I spotted a sign that claimed to mark the spot where the British apprehended hero of the American Revolution, Nathan Hale. I sat and pondered that spot for nearly an hour, trying to picture the scene as it had been nearly two hundred years earlier. At another site, I ventured out behind the model to discover a huge pond, with ducks swimming lazily around in circles. I found some cake in the model, and stayed by the pond feeding it to the ducks.

The adventure of finding the places was enriched by our exploration of the homes themselves. Ranch houses, colonials, split levels, high ceilings, low ceilings, dens and libraries, rec rooms and studies, bare wood floors and carpeting, and on and on the variations went. Mostly, my parents seemed to like all the houses about he same.

What seemed to preoccupy my parents score sheet were things like school systems, access to New York City, financing plans and interest rates. We almost always had either lunch or dinner in the community, especially if we had any interest at all in the homes there. That was my favorite time, partially because I liked to eat, far too much, as a matter of fact, but mostly, because this was the part where we always "took stock" as my father liked to say.

Once we had used the restroom and decided upon our order, the serious conversation would begin. My mother always went first, as she always had a thorough analysis of the advantages and disadvantages of each place. My father would always go next, generally with a host of less than monumental issues, such as prospects for good TV reception, available recreation opportunities, or the potential difficulty of mowing the yard. Then it was our turn, Alan's and mine, and my folks always listened intently, and made us feel as though our opinions were just as important as theirs.

Finally, it all came down to that day in Rockland County, across the Hudson River from New York, in the house with the turned up roof corners, and the romantic name, August Moon Estates. This had not started out to be a good day for house hunting, as I was a bit miffed to be missing the football game that afternoon between the New York Giants and their rivals for the division championship. Initially, I had remained in the car, determined to listen to the game on the car radio. But I could not take my eyes off the faintly Oriental looking home with the lovely little lake nestled against the back yard.

Reluctantly, I had turned off the radio, locked the car, pocketed the keys and slinked up the front walk of the model home. My father smiled to see me, and quickly made his way to my side. He put his arm over my shoulder and asked how the Giants were doing, seeming pleased that they were leading at the half by ten points. By this time, my parents had been sufficiently impressed to progress to stage two: inspection of an actual home that was being built, right next store.

That is how I came to be standing in the rough hewn interior of the house next to the model, somehow enjoying the empty, partially built home even more than the more comfortable model home, perhaps because the idea of our buying a house in the suburbs was suddenly becoming much more real. That January we signed a contract on a lot just a few houses down from the one we had stood in. That day, we had our third of many meals in the Plaza Restaurant in Spring Valley, New York, owned by a local politician, who greeted us and made us feel as though we were already his constituents. The following year we moved into our house in the suburbs, a move that more than lived up to my expectations.

Fairfax County, Virginia June 1996

We had arrived early, David and I, to be sure we arrived at my father's new home before he did. The director of the nursing home greeted us personally, knowing that this was a tough day for us.

Despite my anticipation at seeing Dad and having him close by, the finality of checking him into a full care facility was beginning to sink in. This would be Dad's last new home, though we had no way of knowing for how long.

The nursing home staff had sent someone to pick Dad up at the airport. One of his care providers from Florida had accompanied him for the flight from Ft. Lauderdale, for a fairly reasonable fee. This was the suggested course of action by his doctors, as they felt that being greeted by family upon arrival at the new residence was a good way to initiate his stay there. Had we accompanied him on the trip we would have lost this psychological advantage, since he might no longer know us by the time we arrived in Virginia. So, David and I waited in the front lobby, sitting in comfortable chairs and inhaling the sweet aroma of the fresh flowers, watching for the van to pull up. I found that I looked forward to seeing Dad, though I fretted over how things would go.

Susan and Diana would be arriving soon for additional moral support, and my brother Alan was due for dinner. "Some family reunion," I was thinking. The van pulled up; the nurse got out and helped Dad to his feet on the sidewalk, and suddenly, they were coming toward us through the front door. I moved quickly to intercept them, and hugged my father, who smiled, but seemed a bit dazed. Dad treated me with familiarity, though he thought I was his brother, rather than his son. He was sure that my son, was his son. That was OK…I would settle for him realizing that we were family.

We walked arm in arm toward his new room, smiling, and chatting as best we could about his trip to Virginia. He understood that he was coming to a new place, and that it was nearer to where I lived, though he described the home as a hotel or resort. This was his construct, not a fantasy that we had built. My thoughts floated around, mostly to how and why we had arrived at this moment.

Everyone has an image of what a nursing home is, and it is generally not favorable. We tend to view a nursing home as a place where loved ones go to die…and of course, there is some truth to that notion. A nursing home does tend to be the last stop on the way to the end of life, somewhere that people go out of necessity, not desire. In modern times, this has become increasingly true, as such facilities as senior living quarters and assisted care living have provided halfway stops that can serve older citizens well, giving those who are less than totally dependent an alternative to full care nursing home residence.

As noted earlier, we had tried assisted care living for Dad, and it did not work. Once he left his apartment behind, Dad had descended into the next step down in the Alzheimer's chain, recovering only a little of his senses once he had been there for several weeks. It did no good to wonder whether we could have left Dad in his apartment, since he had become a danger to himself and the cost of keeping him at home with full time care would have been prohibitive (at least four thousand dollars a month), at which rate he would have been bankrupt very quickly, and neither Medicare nor Medicaid would help with this form of care.

The search for a nursing home is not nearly so fun as house hunting, for several obvious, and several not so obvious reasons. The obvious reasons include the sad nature of the reason for the move: when I was a kid we were house hunting, for example, because we could no longer handle living in the city; my wife and I went searching for a nursing home because my father could no longer handle living on his own. What's more: forty years earlier my family would leave behind a small, dark apartment and the sounds of wailing sirens for a spacious home in an idyllic, leafy neighborhood. Now, my father would be giving up an airy assisted care apartment on the beach and the mellow sounds of waves lapping upon the shore, for a darker, institutional home off of a busy highway, with the sounds of old people wailing and coughing.

To be sure, the comparison between house hunting and nursing home selection, leaves little doubt as to which is the happier experience. Nevertheless, the nursing home search was every bit as necessary, still involved my family - this time my wife and kids, God bless them for coming with me - and would still portend a major change in lifestyle for all of us. Though not the delightful adventure of house hunting, the nursing home search still took on the nobility of a family activity, and we strove to make it as pleasant as possible, stopping for lunch in new places, and exploring unfamiliar communities, as feasible. My advice is to work at making it somewhat enjoyable, lest it turn into the nightmare that it can be.

Do not, under any circumstances, be fooled into thinking that you can conduct the search for a nursing home by phone or mail, or by email. While you can do some initial screening by phone or email, you absolutely must visit every serious candidate in person. I suggest visiting all of the candidates, even those you doubt you will select due to extraneous, but important reasons like commuting distance. Every home you visit will give you ideas of what you are looking for, and perhaps just as important, what you are looking to avoid.

You can develop your initial list from several sources. Local agencies on aging will help, and are generally located at the county or city level; they may even have a list already printed that can be picked up, mailed or faxed. In addition, groups such as AARP have resource information on aged care facilities and several magazines that they publish or recommend will often publish listings. You can also contact your local hospital, which may have a sister facility of its own. Last, but not least: ask around. You may be surprised how many of your friends, neighbors and business contacts have aging parents, and many will have recently conducted their own searches. Some lists you obtain may have a mix of different types of facilities, which could include full care options such as nursing homes, and might also have assisted care, seniors living, and everything in between. In this day and age, there are an infinite range of living arrangements available, and you should know what they are, what their requirements and services are and what their costs are.

As a general rule, the higher level of care your parent requires, the higher the cost will be. Retirement villages or senior living may simply be garden or high rise apartments that feature amenities for older persons, bar families with children, and take advantage of public services such as having mass transit available at the front door. These may not cost any more than a normal apartment in your area, and in some jurisdictions, may even enjoy a limited public subsidy that keeps the cost down.

Assisted care, a relatively recent phenomenon of the late twentieth century, can come in all levels of "assistance". In general, these places go for an in-between experience, retaining some of the trappings of private, independent living, while adding some conveniences and safety and health features for those who need a little extra help. For example, assisted care generally means that there is a qualified health professional on the premises at all times, which could be as comprehensive as a nurse on every floor, or as minimal as a lesser practitioner in a central location. Find out exactly what it does mean in each case.

Dining and help with medications is another variable. Most assisted care facilities will have a central dining room or cafeteria. Is this all the place features, or is there assistance available in getting your parent to the dining area? Are special diets catered to? Does anyone keep track of who is showing up for meals regularly and who is not? Is cooking allowed in the individual apartments (not necessarily a plus for forgetful seniors) and is there any provision for catered dining to the individual apartments?

Most seniors, particularly those with dementia problems, are on medication, more often than not, a whole rainbow of medications. Can the facility handle dispensing of meds, or do they just offer help when it is requested? Some simply check in with residents periodically to ask whether they have taken their meds, while others check up more rigorously. This is something that you should not have to worry over once your parent is in assisted care if you choose the right place; forgetting to take medicines regularly is one of the things that put many seniors in a facility in the first place, and one cannot overestimate the importance of predictability in dosing medications for seniors.

The nursing home is an ultimate solution, one that implies total care. It is invariably a long-term care facility, which must include a qualified medical staff, the ability to give both routine and special medications, full service residential and medical care and a means for addressing emergency situations. It is the residence of last resort, where, as one callous rep for a nursing home that we did not choose told me, "the only way that residents leave is to die." A case in point: can you guess why we did not choose that particular nursing home?

Harsh as this comment may seem…it is all too true. Which does not make it any easier to engage in the search for a nursing home.

Whether your parent is at that residence of last resort stage or not, you would do well to study the differences in what each of the various levels of elder care provide. One resource that you have which was not always available in the past, is the Internet. As with so many topics, the Internet has become a powerful tool for people searching out different alternatives for elder care. There are websites that can help you with all of the various aspects of this exercise. You might do well to start with an exploration of the stages of care descriptions and then progress to using the Internet to find actual facilities in your area. I am not going to recommend specific websites, as the availability of sites changes almost daily. Choose a good search engine and put in key words like "seniors" or "elderly housing", or better yet, "assisted care" or "nursing home", and a myriad of choices will be instantly in front of you.

I will steer you toward the websites on Medicare and Medicaid, since understanding these programs and their use is a central issue for most of us in making arrangements for our elder parents. Try www.medicare.gov and www.hcfa.gov/medicaid/medicaid.htm for information on both programs. Unless you are more than independently wealthy, you will want to know how these two resources work, what their limitations are, how to utilize them, and just as important, how they differ. I will attempt only the briefest of tips here, and refer you to their respective US Government websites for more details.

In short, Medicare is a health insurance program administered by the federal government, and intended for the elderly and disabled. It will cover finite hospital stays (Part A) and medical treatments (Part B). For the most part, the hospital coverage is free, as you have probably been paying into Medicare your whole life from paycheck withholding. The medical insurance (Part B) generally costs a nominal fee (like $50/month). Many seniors opt to use Medicare Part B for their primary health insurance due to its reasonable cost and relative ease of use. However, take note: coverage is limited, and most seniors who can afford it opt to take out additional health insurance, often referred to as a "Medicare Supplement", to pick up the things and portions of bills not covered under Medicare. Many companies can be used for this purpose, and the cost is not generally prohibitive.

Do not confuse the Medicare Part A coverage with that of Medicaid, which is a joint federal-state administered program for Long Term Care. This is invoked in the case of those elderly and disabled persons who must have full time long-term care and cannot afford it. While Medicare Part A does include some nursing home coverage, it is not intended to pay for lifelong care for the resident. Medicaid does…but you had better know your stuff regarding its rules and regulations

The good news is that under Medicaid, there is no reason why any deserving older person cannot afford quality, long-term care in a fine facility. That should help you sleep at night. However, as would seem only fair, the government is going to pick up the full cost of elder care, only for those who truly need the assistance. Fair as that seems, the intricacies of determining who does and who does not really need this financial help has created a cottage industry for government workers and elder care attorneys. I do not mean to seem crass here: many of these individuals are quite innocent of blame for this quagmire, and in fact, often hate it as much as you may come to.

The problem of course, is that only the indigent truly have NO MONEY at all. Everyone else has some resources. What's more, many senior citizens have only their modest savings accounts to show for a lifetime of hard work and paying taxes, and would very much like to hold on to some portion and even pass a bit along to their children. Technically, every penny of your parent's money must be expended before he or she can use Medicaid to pay for their long-term care. This is the tricky part.

Make no mistake: on the one hand, there are perfectly legal ways in which a very limited share of your parent's money can be passed along to his heirs, and still qualify for Medicaid. On the other hand: the rules regarding how much this is and how and when it may be disposed of, are strict, complicated and changing all the time. Be aware that an aging parent in need of long-term care cannot, under any circumstances, simply give you and other heirs all his money, and then merrily apply for Medicaid to cover his living expenses.

Your best bet is to find out NOW what the federal and state regulations are regarding how much money can be given away and when that can be done in relation to the time when Medicaid is applied for. There are volume limits, and timing restrictions. If your parent gives away too much money too close to the time when he/she applies for Medicaid coverage, even by one day, the penalties in terms of delays in eligibility are swift and severe. This could well be the cause of your parent no longer having his own resources and not being covered by Medicaid to cover his long-term care, so be wary.

Get used to the idea that money management is now, unless you have more money than you know what to do with, a major element in deciding on your parent's housing. Keep in mind that it will cost one of you anywhere from $2,000 to $5,000 to as much as $10,000 per month to keep your parent housed in a safe and supportive environment. You can also keep up with costs by surfing the Internet for information, but whatever you find, it will inevitably mean an annual bill large enough to equal a nice living for someone. Even for people of substantial means, this is going to be a big bite, one that may eventually leave your loved one in need of financial assistance.

My advice: obtain the services of a good elder care attorney, and if necessary, one who specializes in Medicaid use and eligibility. I used a total of three attorneys: an elder care/estate attorney in my father's home state, an experienced estate attorney in my state, and a Medicaid specialist in my state. They were well worth it.

Medicaid also has different rules and cost allowances from state to state, so an expert on YOUR state, the state where your parent will be domiciled, is essential.

Now you get into yet another variable: the variations in the way that nursing homes handle Medicaid patients. The need to check this out simply blends into the overall list of things to look for in a nursing home, so we will return to that exercise.

Here are some questions you might ask, even before you visit the nursing home:

-What is the monthly cost, including extras such as laundry, special diet needs, administering medications, etc?

-What provision does the facility make for medical care in the case of seriously ill patients?

-Is there a special program for dementia patients and are they separated from the general population?

-Does the home accept Medicaid patients, and are they separated from the general population?

-What happens in the case of someone who enters the facility with their own resources, but is forced to apply for Medicaid coverage because their money has run out?

-Does the home have staff will can assist you in understanding and applying for Medicaid, or are you on your own?

-Is the home affiliated with any assisted care or other forms of progressive care facilities, in case your parent is not yet ready for a nursing home?

-If you are actually placing your parent in an affiliated assisted care facility, how seamless is the progression from assisted care to the full care nursing home? Is admission guaranteed when it is time to move up, or are you on the waiting list along with everyone else?

-If you are not yet ready to make the move, what is the general waiting period for an opening? If you are ready, same question.

-Availability of amenities such as public transportation, basic shopping, nearest hospital...these are for YOUR convenience.

In every case there should be someone at the home who can answer these questions, generally the admissions director. If not, scratch the place off your list. In our case, there was a nursing home that would have been very desirable in terms of location, but three phone calls failed to get me someone who could answer these questions. I took this as a bad sign. In another case, the person I did get on the phone was impatient and quite rude (that was the woman who told me that the only way people left, to create openings, was to die). Again, a bad sign.

If personnel at the home seem incompetent, impatient, unhelpful or rude now, just wait until they have your parent as a resident and are really teed off at your insistent demands and your parent's cranky complaints.

A note on long-term care insurance: Offered under several different names, this relatively new option refers to private insurance, which is purchased ahead of the need, that will cover the cost associated with long-term care. It is expensive…there is no other way to put it. But it will guarantee that the purchaser can pay for long-term residence in a nursing home; that his assets will be protected for his heirs; and that no government aid will be needed.

The Visit

OK…so now we get to the "fun", house hunting part of finding a nursing home. You and your spouse get up early and get spruced up; you leave the house clutching your list of places and the directions to each one. Next to each place on the list is the name of your contact in admissions, and maybe a few of your notes from your research and the phone conversation.

You make your approach and start sizing up the place from the outside. It's all right to start sizing things up, it's what you're there for. Pay attention to what the place looks like, how it sounds, what it smells like. These are the sensations that your parent will be living with, so don't overlook anything. Don't limit your visit to the office, or even a few main rooms; you must take the full tour: see the patient rooms, the dining area, and all recreation facilities. Pay attention to how the residents look and behave: are they clean? Do they smile at all? Are they talking to each other and the staff?

Meet all the staff you can. These are the people that will make up your parent's world and they cannot all fake it. What is the lighting like? Are there plenty of windows and light? What is the view like? What about security: is it adequate, without being prison-like? Do the residents wear tracking badges or bracelets, or does the facility depend solely on locked doors?

Then there is the remaining factor: intangibles. Are there fresh flowers around? Does anyone ever come in with entertainment, puppies, counseling, religious services or special treats for the residents? The nursing home we picked had flowers, birds in cages and a resident golden retriever. If you are seriously interested, but still unsure, consider dropping in on all the finalist facilities, unannounced. Go in and wander around to see how things appear on an unguided, unguarded tour. This is something that you MUST do after you pick the place to make sure that you really know how well your parent is being treated.

No matter how much you like a facility, you will not be able to recapture the feeling of buying that special new home. But, under the right circumstances, the right place will give you a feeling of peace and security. It is after all, the answer to your parent's difficult situation. And, if you are lucky enough to be looking at assisted care because your parent still just needs a little supervision to make sure he eats and takes his medicine, then the place may be quite lovely. My father's brief stay in assisted care was in a high rise Marriott facility on the beach in Ft. Lauderdale…a place my son said he would not have minded living in.

For assisted care, don't forget to find out about the level of assisted care, check on the availability of transportation to shopping, the types of recreational facilities and the availability of progressive care, for later on.

Try not to let the nursing home search depress you. Once you adjust to it, and this means you, as well as your parent, the nursing home does not have to be a totally unpleasant experience, in fact, it should not be. Remember that this is your parent's new place to live, it isn't a funeral. But trust your instincts; if the place depresses you, it is probably not the right one for your parent.

Chapter Eight

The Credit Card...Don't Leave Home With It

Nanuet, New York, October 1964: The Gloved One

Even at fourteen, a near miss in the finals of the league championship series really hurt. And it was all my fault. At least it felt that way, on a gray, chilly October Monday, with the smell of hot dogs and freshly cut grass still mingled with tears that were creeping down my cheeks.

I had done something in the championship game that had never been much a part of my repertoire: I had missed an easy play on the horsehide, the baseball, and that miss had opened the floodgates for the other team to stage a remarkable comeback and beat us in the final inning for the championship. I had no explanation. I had just missed the routine play on the ball, no excuses. I thought that was only a little deal at that moment, but my play would have been the third out, the final out of the game. Instead, the other team scored three runs, with two outs, to win by one. The post game team meeting had been a mostly silent one, and I had at least appreciated the fact that my manager and teammates had done nothing but console me, reminding me that no one play had won or lost a championship, and that nothing could take away from the great season that we had all experienced.

The kindness of my team and coaches only made it worse. So my father had kept quiet, thus far, sensing my pain, and knowing that words might only hurt more than the silence. He didn't have to tell me that it was OK with him, and that he was proud of me; I knew these things without hearing them, such was the nature of my father, and the security I felt in our relationship. Words were unnecessary.

I noticed that rain had started to fall, and wished the rain had started about two hours earlier, so that the last few innings of our game would have been washed out. I also realized, suddenly, that we were not making the turn for home, but were heading in a different direction. Puzzled, I looked over at my Dad in the driver's seat. Sensing my confusion, he finally spoke.

"Would you mind taking a few minutes to run an errand. I need to stop off at the store for a minute?"

I just nodded, numbly, that I was OK with that plan.

Dad eased the car into the relative quiet of the parking lot of my favorite department store. E.J. Korvette was one of the first of the "super stores", carrying everything from household items to electronics to sporting goods. It was a massive building, with gray brick siding and lots of glass, and a sign that stood twenty feet high in bold red script. Rumor had it that the chain had been started by a group of Eight Jewish Korean (War) Veterans, and that the name was an acronym that had been drawn from this unusual grouping of founders.

I hoped we would not have to be there too long.

Before I could tell Dad that I would wait in the car, he asked me to come in and help him pick something out. I figured it was to be something for the house, and that my mother was so particular, that he needed me for advice and validation. I agree to help.

We entered the brightly lit fluorescence of E.J. Kovette, and my attention was naturally drawn over to the right where the huge sporting goods department sat invitingly. Much to my surprise, my father was already over at the tall display that featured about two hundred baseball gloves, smelling of leather and opportunity. Dad was pounding his fist into one glove just now, a sly smile playing across his face.

"I thought it might be time for a new glove. You know your hands have grown so much in the last year, and that old Tony Kubek model may just be a bit small. You never know when that old glove might not be long enough to reach an important hit. Wanna try one on?"

I couldn't believe my ears. I had been lobbying for a new glove all season, but had known in my heart that the old one was fine. So what if I had been using that old Kubek model since I was ten years old? It was fine, if a bit small, but that had been the style that the big leaguers favored in my father's day. Only in the 1960s had the new, larger glove designs become more popular with the pros and with kids.

Dad handed me the glove he had tried on. It was an Al Kaline model, nice, but not quite the one I had been looking at all season. Gloves loomed enticingly from metal hooks in the pegboard on the display, all with new leather smell and pockets waiting to be pounded. And then, there was the glove of my dreams: the new Rawlings Rocky Colavito model. Rocky was a great home run hitter who played for Cleveland and Detroit, a man's man, who every Yankee fan like myself admired and coveted for our Yankees. He was as Italian as they come, and there had always been an affinity between Italians and Jews in the Bronx, at least among my friends and neighbors, so we considered Rocky to be one of our own.

My father knew most of this; I suspect now that he knew all along just which glove I had been pining for all this time, though I had never told him. I slipped it over my hand, wondering what Dad would think. I already knew it would be perfect.

The fit could not have been better, just as it had been during a few trial runs when I had snuck into this department before during previous trips with my mother. But this was different. Putting the glove on my hand, while my Dad watched, and with a chance to perhaps really buy the beauty...this was entirely different. Then I saw the price; this one was, by twenty dollars, the most expensive glove in the entire store. I knew we would not be getting the Rocky Colavito model. Without a word, I slipped it off and started trying on other gloves. Something else would surely make do; there were similar models with less cost attached.

Dad watched me, while still trying on more gloves himself.

"You know, I like that Colavito. Didn't you?"

I was stunned.

"But, Dad, what about the price? I thought the price was a little steep."

He smiled, not just with his mouth, but with his whole face, the way only my Dad could. There was something about his eyebrows that completed my Dad's bigger smiles, just as they did at that magic moment.

"If that glove is the perfect one, not just good, but perfect, then we can get it. Hey, isn't that what a credit card is for?"

"What will Mom say, Dad?"

"She would see things exactly the same way. So, is that the perfect glove, or not?"

I hugged my Dad, by way of an answer. He already knew.

A few wonderful minutes later we had found the register and Dad was pulling out his credit card. The clerk seemed to take years to call in the purchase and to put Rocky Colavito in the bag for me. The glove was on my hand before we had cleared the front door. I didn't take Rocky Colavito off for three days, even at school.

Over the next week, all I could think about was that glove. I oiled it, I worked the pocket, I stuffed a baseball into the pocket and tied the glove around the ball to soften and deepen the pocket. I slept with the glove either in my arms, or under my pillow. And I dreamed of next season, wishing that spring baseball could start right now. I completely forgot that only a few short days ago I had never wanted to play baseball again.

That had not been a good year for championships in my world; my beloved Yankees lost a heart breaking World Series to the St. Louis Cardinals in 1964, ending one of the longest runs of success of any team in any sport. They did not appear in the World Series again until the late 1970s.

But my fiercest memory from the Fall of 1964, superseding all others, was that early evening trip to E.J. Korvette, and the feeling of pure euphoria that lodged in my brain and my stomach, the moment I knew that the Rocky Colavito glove might be mine, and stayed with me for months. Did I say months…I mean years; that feeling is as alive within me today, nearly forty years later, as it was the day we bought "Rocky". That was the name my famous glove took on, after the ballplayer who lent his name to its manufacture.

Over the years I have played adult softball and even a little baseball with Rocky on my hand. Back in the early 1980s the leather bindings that held Rocky together began to wear out and snap, one by one. I played on with the glove as best I could. During the winter that year, Rocky mysteriously disappeared. He had finally come completely undone during a late season game at shortstop, when a pretty little snag of a screaming line drive had caused Rocky's final strings to pop, as if the glove had been exploded from within.

Before I could complete the painful chore of shopping for a new glove, Rocky reappeared on my birthday that next April. My wife and brother had found a leather craftsman, who had been able to reconstruct Rocky, good as new. Since then I have taught my own son to play baseball, with Rocky on my hand, and have taken Rocky to many more major league games with us, hoping to catch a foul ball. Just like when I was a kid, going to Yankee Stadium with my Dad.

My best time with Rocky may well have been the day that David's own glove came apart during a little league game, and he asked if he could borrow Rocky for the rest of the game. I was thrilled to comply, and Rocky finished out that season on my son's hand. When the season ended, we went shopping for a new glove. Wouldn't you know that David picked out a glove that was the spitting image of Rocky. His grandfather would have been proud.

I have Rocky to this day, well preserved and cared for. I have the memory, too, of that trip to the store with my Dad, and the sweet little trick he pulled to turn my worst day in baseball into one of my very best. And he accomplished his little miracle with a simple flip of that piece of plastic, the trusty credit card.

Manassas, Virginia October, 1996

It was an unseasonably warm evening, and we had opened the back door to allow the warm fall breeze to waft through the kitchen. The kids sat at the kitchen table carving their pumpkins, as I tried to supervise, but not interfere too much. These were among the first jack-o-lanterns that I had let them carve themselves, with knives that were short, but sharp. At twelve and ten I figured they were old enough. We were in high spirits, and Susan had a pie baking in the oven.

David's baseball uniform lay along the kitchen floor, where he had unceremoniously stripped it off and discarded it, piece by piece. We had only been home a short time, having just gotten home from a ballgame under the lights. Although not the final game, this had been a win in the second round of the fall playoffs, the farthest we had gotten in several years. The team I coached, my David's team, had beaten the heavy favorite, a team that had beaten us badly in the regular season. My son had played competently, solid as always on defense, and two for four at bat. We had all had hot dogs at the game, so dinner was not an issue.

I looked fondly at David's glove (the one so much like Rocky) laying quietly on the kitchen chair, and thought of that day so many years ago when my Dad had taken me to buy my glove. Then the phone rang.

A male voice asked for my father. When I explained who I was he went on to say that it did not matter who I was, that I owed money to his bank for credit card debts incurred by my father. I reiterated that I was the son, not the father, and told him that my father had Alzheimer's and was in a nursing home.

Here is how he responded:

"Well, that's not my fault. You still owe the money!!!"

I told him that I was not legally responsible for my father's debts, and he said that somebody was, and that we had better pay up.

I asked if he had heard me say that my father had Alzheimer's. Here is how he responded:

"Oh, boo hoo. Like I had anything to do with that, or care. What do you want me to do about it? You better pay this bill. You and your father can't just weasel out of this bill, just because he got sick. You better take care of this, or you will be sorry, both of you."

I suggested that he go visit Dad in the nursing home and see what he could get out of him. Here is how he responded:

"I might just do that. If he's in a nursing home, someone must be paying for it. They cost a lot of money, and I'll find out how to get at it." Here is how I responded:

"Like Hell you will, you coldhearted SOB."

To which he had the nerve to say, "So, now you're going to get nasty?"

I hung up, cursing. It was time to turn these people over to our lawyer.

The trusty credit card had not been so trustworthy for my father in his later years. Of course he thought it was; he loved his credit cards, and showed it by giving them a workout regularly, and by allowing them to go visiting from time to time. In the two years preceding my father's ultimate move into the nursing home, he ran up at least fifty thousand dollars in credit card debt. This was accomplished with the help of at least six different credit cards, and the ease of using these cards without benefit of a valid signature.

My advice: take away all credit cards and tear them up, just as soon as you suspect your father is not fully cognizant. He will buy things on impulse; he will buy them over the phone, and through the television. He will lend out his credit card, give it to someone to make a purchase on his behalf, or give it to someone to "buy their own birthday present". He will trust someone with the card to buy his groceries or pay his bills, or to get him cash. And…you cannot be sure of anyone's honesty; the temptation is simply too great. The friends, neighbors, caregivers, cleaning people and strangers who will get their hands on his credit card and use that card liberally, will surprise you.

Part of the problem in dealing with Dad's credit card bills was that you could not determine: how much he incurred when in his right mind; how much he incurred, but without understanding what he was doing; how much was run up by people who knew Dad in some capacity; how much was run up by people who somehow got hold of his credit card numbers; and how much was simply wrong. Compounding the problem were the numerous interest charges, late payment penalties and annual fees. There was no way to determine whether any of these were being applied to legitimate charges.

Herein lies the crux of the matter: what does constitute a legitimate charge? If Dad himself incurred a given charge, how to determine what his state of mind was at the time, and to figure out whether it mattered, legally, what condition he was in. Furthermore, if a charge was incurred by a friend, neighbor, or caregiver, but they were doing so under instructions from my father, who was responsible for the charge?

From the point of view of the credit card companies and the banks that administer bankcards - VISA and MasterCard, for example - the charges are all legitimate and must be paid. After all, they would maintain that, if Dad were not in his right mind, we could have canceled the cards. This was easier said than done for two reasons: 1) We were a little slow to know when Dad eased over the line mentally, and he was resistant to giving up his credit cards and 2) We never did even find many of Dad's credit cards nor any record of their bills. We could only address the status of cards or bills we could find, and even that was often difficult, as most credit card companies won't let anyone other than the authorized user cancel the card.

I did not become fully aware of the extent of Dad's credit card fiasco until my address and phone number began to get associated with Dad's affairs. Somehow, even though Dad never lived in my house for any length of time, the credit cards, and other creditors, found me. Once they did, many of them did all they could to make my life a living Hell. Whether dealing with the collections department from the credit card company, or the collections bureaus they engaged, I learned what it must be like to be insolvent.

Here are a few of my favorite illustrations:

· Bill collectors would call very early in the morning (as early as six a.m., and very late at night (as late as eleven p.m.)

· Bill collectors would call on weekends and holidays

· Bill collectors would somehow get my phone number at work, call me at the office, and often would abuse whoever answered the phone at the office

· Bill collectors would call, and if one of my children or my wife would answer the phone, would abuse and/or threaten them

· Bill collectors would abuse me, threaten me, try to trick me, would hang up and call right back, would yell at me

· Bill collectors would offer settlement deals, but would say the deals had a limited shelf life

· Bill collectors would sometimes call every day for weeks, often professing not to know that the same company had already called

These are the tip of the iceberg. The collectors would tell me that they would come after me and would ruin my credit. They said that they would visit my father at the nursing home and would search for assets - I told them to go right ahead. I would talk to someone from a credit card company who seemed totally reasonable, only to find that they would refer me from one department to another, with no one able to bring things to a resolution. I would have a rare good call with one of the credit card company representatives, only to get a call from a different rep the very next day, and this person would claim to have no knowledge nor any record of my earlier conversation.

The initial position of virtually every company was basically that Dad owed the money, that there would be no deal, but that we could make arrangements for a repayment schedule. My position was that I was questioning all charges, based on my father's impaired capacity and the fact that some of the cards were missing and presumed stolen. In at least one case, I know the charges to be fraudulent, since the charges were for gasoline, and Dad's car had been taken away months before. Some of the credit card companies were, or appeared to be, sympathetic, though this did not always make any difference in how we proceeded. In some cases, the companies had established, formal procedures for questioning charges in a case like this. Others had procedures, but not tailored to our particular situation. Some had entirely separate departments that handled these kinds of cases, and we were turned over to those departments, though collections people would still often call.

Your first issue is to know what your legal position, not just your moral position, is. I had one big thing going for me: I was not in any way legally responsible for Dad's debts. Rarely would a child or sibling have legal responsibility for the patient's debts unless they had arranged to do so. Thus, I had some leverage, in that I was talking to these companies out of the goodness of my heart, not out of any legal necessity. They could threaten to ruin Dad's credit, which was fine with me, but even that was a fairly empty threat. There were, of course, some of Dad's resources to protect. Though by no means a fortune, they would cover his care for a while, if we could manage them carefully.

The second issue revolves around what recourse you have for bills that need to be questioned or challenged. Several of the credit card companies were nice enough to tell me that we would not be responsible for any bills that were incurred by Dad when he had Alzheimer's. Most admitted that they could not collect for bills incurred by other people using Dad's cards or numbers. The problem in both cases, was how to establish which bills were not "legitimate". I was confused about the timing of the charges and how to make even a reasonable guess as to which bills really should be paid. Above all, I wondered who had the burden of proof.

A very few companies were especially cooperative. In two cases, one a bankcard, and one a credit card, the companies asked me if I could document the onset of the dementia. I explained what little I could do to prove his early problems, and they asked if I would be willing to pay all charges incurred prior to the documented onset of dementia. That seemed very reasonable, and so we settled pretty quickly. I asked them to send current statements, went through the bills and found a reasonable date to use as a cutoff. Those two companies then forgave the later charges, with no further questions asked. My only mistake was that I should have insisted on a more formal signed agreement confirming that these accounts were settled in full. The bank card would become a problem a year later, when the bank that had been so nice was taken over by another bank that was considerably less friendly. The nicest, most reasonable and most cooperative company I dealt with was a credit card company who shall remain nameless; but I have not left home without that company's credit card since.

Some of the credit card companies would assign a case officer to work with me on determining the validity of the charges. In these cases, many phone calls were exchanged and mountains of paper arrived at my home. I wanted to see monthly statements, and also requested signed credit card receipts, with mixed success. Many hours were spent trying to verify charges and the nature of those charges.

I decided after a while that some of the companies had no desire to "rip off" an aging Alzheimer's patient or his suffering family. To varying degrees, these companies were working with me to try to find a reasonable figure to settle upon, while suspending the accumulation of interest and late charges. In several cases, we found a mutually satisfactory middle ground, and I paid them off. Unfortunately, for some of these companies, the fact that I was working with their reps to resolve things did not stop people from some other department from calling to harass me. In other cases, even after I thought we had reached an agreement, the company or their hired bill collector came back after me later on.

In general, I simply refused to acknowledge any charges that were incurred over the phone. I challenged any charges that had been incurred after my visit to Florida during which I had taken away Dad's car. As the process dragged on for the better part of a year, the calls and harassment began to get to me. I also was sick of the companies who reneged on the deals I thought we had reached.

The October evening phone call described earlier had been the last straw, and I brought in our lawyer. At his advice, I had been trying to handle all I could on my own, to save money, but this had gone far enough. I did not need legal protection, but my sanity was suffering.

The attorney made his first priority a cessation of the harassment. He wrote to all the credit card companies who had been calling and told them that: 1) the phone calls must stop, or they would be reported to the state attorney general for prosecution under Virginia laws that protect debtors from harassment; 2) that I was not legally responsible for my father's debts and was talking to them out of sheer good will, which they should appreciate and reflect in their dealings with me; 3) that my father suffered from severe dementia, and had for some time, and thus we were challenging all credit card charges; and 4) that they could supply signed receipts for all charges and we would consider paying charges that had been so documented.

The calls slowed to a trickle, almost immediately. Within a month virtually every company had made a settlement offer. My attorney said I had several choices.

· I could continue to challenge all charges. The problem here was that the credit card companies were unlikely to go away, and might continue to press for full payment, past the point where my father's resources had run out or could be exhausted by the credit card claims. They might forget about us for a while, and resurface years later. It was murky as to what their recourse, or mine, would be at that point.

· I could agree to the settlement offers.

· I could make counter offers that we deemed reasonable.

We decided to make counter offers to all those who had responded - not every company chose to acknowledge the attorney's letter.

In every case, they eventually settled, mostly on the terms we had proposed, which ranged from twenty-five to fifty cents on the dollar. We insisted upon a signed letter that declared all debt settled in full. This ended most of the problems with credit card companies, although one has just come out of the woodwork, some five years later, and stubbornly continues to call and write, in spite of my written documentation. They say that they are going to ruin Dad's credit; I tell them to go right ahead!

You will never look at credit cards the same way again.

Chapter Nine

Make the Hard Decisions...Before They Become Impossible

It's time to buckle down and tell you about the rest of the things you simply must do. These are lessons learned from dealing with an Alzheimer's patient, but they apply to most of our aging parents, regardless of what name you put on the disease. I have had to serve as Executor for an unmarried uncle, who died rather suddenly, of a heart attack, and many of the same issues applied. Likewise, I have found myself counseling several friends with aging parents, some with Alzheimer's, some with other diseases, and some with no real diagnosis, other than aging, and again, the issues are strikingly similar.

It's Not Crass to Put Finances High on Your List

Most of us consider managing our own money to be enough of a challenge, without taking responsibility for someone else's. In addition, no aging parent likes to give up control of his/her money, due to some extent to the mistrust of others, warranted or otherwise, and partly due to independence issues. Money, as much or more than any other factor in their lives, is central to their self-view as adult, independent, functioning human beings, and the loss of control strikes many seniors as tantamount to throwing in the towel. We've already covered their desire to hang onto credit cards, and the disastrous consequences that can ensue. Of course, we owe it to our aging parents to respect their dignity and to find every way possible to allow them some retention of money control. In traditional households, this can be tougher to deal with when men are involved, regardless of whether they actually handled the finances in their married household. Nevertheless, I have seen cases of both men and women who stubbornly cling to the perception of control over their finances, even when they have no background in managing their own money.

Indeed, the most difficult senior to deal with can often be the one who had always depended on a spouse to manage the money, has no idea how to do it, but is loathe to cede this function to an adult child. My father had taken to becoming very literal with money, even though, during my mother's management regime he had rarely had anything to do with finances, other than having some cash and credit cards in his wallet.

Of course, this was the very thing we had taken away from him. No more credit cards, no checkbook, and precious little cash, if any. So there he would be, with no visible signs of currency, and it frustrated him, worse still, it frightened him.

One evening Susan and I returned from dinner out with the kids and amidst the jovial good spirits of a happy family with full stomachs, we turned on the answering machine to hear our messages. The first one froze me in my tracks.

"Miles, this is your father…it's Dad. I don't know what to do…I'm desperate for money, you must help me." His voice was frail and wavering badly. The message went on, after a pause.

"You have taken away all my cash and credit cards, I have no checkbook and no way to get money or to buy food. I don't know how I will live; you must help me. Please call me tonight, because I'm afraid that I'll starve to death if you don't send me some money…I don't know what to do, and I'm desperate…"

Can you imagine how this call made me feel? I called Dad back immediately and explained that his caregivers had access to money to buy him food, and that I would be paying his bills. I reminded him as to why he did not have money, credit cards or a checkbook, though I did it gently. That call from my father was to be repeated many times. The calls only stopped when he ceased to understand even what money was.

Ironically, the aging senior is often able to hold on only to the perception of control, because the unreliability of his/her mind makes control over money a slippery illusion. For the Alzheimer's patient, the one in control of your father's money is not your father, but the seriously altered state of his mind. To put it another way, it would be as if an alien had inhabited your father's body, and took control of his mind, either from time to time, or full time. This alien gradually assumes full control over dad's finances, while allowing dad the illusion of control. It is insidious, but as certain as the sun coming up in the morning, which, in itself, becomes a tricky concept for the patient.

This may seem radical, but in fact there is nothing to prepare you for the altered perception your father will have about money, and the awful choices he will inevitably make. This is not about an aging parent simply selling that piece of land you wanted him to keep, or in fact keeping sentimental possessions that you think could well be disposed of. Your father isn't just forgetting things, or losing a sense of perspective...you must get it into your head that your father is NOT your father any more! His entire perception of the world is now skewed, and not always in the same way. Imagine him as being on mind-altering drugs, which make tables look like cruise ships and umbrellas look like snakes. Salesmen appear to your father as his minister or rabbi, and the microwave is his neighbor, Sam. I am not exaggerating. Let me illustrate.

My father sold his house and moved into an apartment. He placed all of the proceeds of his house sale in his regular checking account. Every month he saw a huge balance in his checking account, eventually losing site of the fact that the balance represented his house sale, and thinking instead that the money was from investments, salary or some other form of earning. He was using his checkbook, and was with it enough to see that he always had money left over at the end of the month, so he deluded himself into thinking that he was making more than he was spending.

Every month, my father wrote checks for several thousand dollars. Some were to pay legitimate bills, but many were not. He was also donating a small fortune to charities - most of them legitimate - was entering numerous sweepstakes, each with a small entry fee and was also investing money in a variety of ventures.

Furthermore, my father was giving cash to a variety of individuals as loans or investments, was also giving them cash to shop for him. In several instances, my father gave cash to people he trusted to buy Christmas presents for his grandchildren, or to go to the grocery store. Naturally, there was never any kind of accounting for any of these cash transactions. Any smooth talking stranger who knocked on the door, or called on the phone was likely to come away with cash or a check.

My father ran through roughly $100,000 in just over one year; as best I can tell, about two thirds of it was unnecessary. Something to check on: if you have made proper arrangements to protect your father's money but his bank still cashes and honors his checks, it is possible that the bank may have some liability. So...stay on top of this.

How could it come to this? How could we allow him to do it? Well...you have to remember that my father, at that time, still appeared completely lucid, most of the time. He had what appeared to be memory lapses, and at times, seemed a little confused, but aren't these things normal for aging parents? His apartment was always clean, because he had someone coming in; he could handle a telephone and we talked several times every week; he was still driving for most of that time; his bills were always, or almost always, paid; and he could carry on an intelligent conversation about politics, literature, and other abstract topics. So...how was I to know that he was liquidating virtually all of his assets and allowing his nest egg to be dissipated? Likewise, he could fool people at the bank or just about anywhere else. And his popularity at the bank, after years of building warm, easygoing relationships, made the tellers and managers inclined to respond to most of his seemingly reasonable requests.

I finally insisted on seeing my father's checkbook on my trip to Florida after his fender bender. My father's confusion immediately after the very minor accident - having passed out from a fever, after forgetting to take his antibiotics - and the concern of his girlfriend led me to believe that I needed to look more closely into his lifestyle. I was, naturally, appalled. Yet, even at that stage, I had to steal dad's checkbook while he was sleeping, in order to look at the details of his current finances. He wanted no prying from me, and certainly had no intention of turning over his finances.

Every suggestion that he let me, or my brother help him manage his money elicited protests, and eventually, accusations of greed. Suddenly, I was faced with the reality that my father had squandered his safety net, and might well come to an inglorious end as an indigent. My brother and I make comfortable livings, but we both have children of our own, and were in no position to assume the substantial cost of supporting a parent who needed special care. Thus, it was imperative that we seize control of dad's finances.

Now there are two ways this can be done, the easy way and the hard way. The easy way is to reach some kind of arrangement with your parent when he is still lucid and has some degree of understanding of what is going on. They may fight you, but they will have a better chance of arranging things the way THEY want them, and it will be so much easier for you. Wills can be drawn up, trusts established, powers of attorney signed, joint bank accounts set up, etc. A living trust will gain you some control of the situation, and can be set up 'for the benefit of' (FBO) your parent. You can have sole control, the best idea, make your parent a trustee, add any appropriate relatives you need to or turn to someone outside the family. My advice: keep the number of trustees as small as you can, and do not let the patient have the ability to write checks or withdraw money on his or her own.

A living trust will also allow you to bypass probate when your parent passes on, and can be maintained as a money management tool indefinitely, if you wish.

As you may recall, this was the fortunate route we followed, more or less. As described earlier, I'm not sure we could have pulled it off without Dad's girlfriend, who was a positive, trusted influence and had led the way by example.

A much less pleasant route to take is to wait until your parent has completely lost any ability to function. To some of you, this may seem like the easy way out. Waiting your stubborn, suspicious, combative Dad out may seem simple, appealing. Then they probably will not be able to fight you, but there may be little or no money left to fight over. At this point, you must prepare a case to have your parent declared incompetent and have yourself (or another) appointed as a guardian. This is not a lot of fun, nor terribly efficient, since you may be closing the barn door after the horse has left.

To reiterate the path we took: we were determined to try the easy way. We started with long talks, over the course of several days. Still, Dad resisted. His girl friend came to the rescue, God bless her. She had (as mentioned earlier) long ago established a Living Trust, which her son had control of, and was very pleased with the way it worked. She also loved the security of knowing that, if and when she lost full control of her senses, her trusted son would at least be able to care for her, with her own money. She persuaded my father to work with me to find a solution that worked. She also persuaded me to find an attorney who could work with me and with my father. At that point, I had found the qualified, sympathetic elder care attorney described earlier, and she was instrumental in making things work. She worked with Dad in a way that reassured him that he was arranging things in the way that HE wanted them. She allowed my father to be the arbiter of the arrangement, but with her guidance as to what made sense from a legal point of view. My father had agreed to meet with the attorney on the condition that his girlfriend could participate, and have a voice. I supported that idea and removed myself from the equation.

All takes time, however, and I was afraid that my father would be penniless by the time we got a trust set up. Fortunately, most of his remaining assets were in mutual funds, through a broker. We took two approaches: first, dad's girl friend agreed to have him live with her, temporarily, both for his safety and to keep him away from his bank and broker, so that he could not divest himself of any more funds. We then got him to agree to add my name to one of his bank accounts, transferring enough money into that account to pay his bills for a few months, and hiding away his other checkbook. I left for home, feeling somewhat at ease that we had, at least, stopped the bleeding, and looking forward to hearing about his meeting with the attorney.

Unfortunately, I had underestimated both Dad's dementia and his determination. Less than a week after I got home, Dad's banker, with whom I had visited while in Florida, called with bad news. Somehow Dad had gotten to the bank and had written a check, drawing out nearly all of the money from the joint account we were going to use to pay his bills. The bank had been alerted to Dad's problem, and was supposed to watch for this kind of thing...but a young teller, who knew and liked dad, and had not gotten the message, went ahead and cashed the check for him, somehow. In spite of all my careful preparations, Dad had now lost several thousand dollars more. And lost is the precise word: no one ever found out what dad did with that money!

The worst part, in some sense, is that gaining control of Dad's finances was no victory. There were, first and foremost, incredible challenges just in terms of money management. But what I never saw coming was just how devastated and terrified Dad would become over having absolutely no discretionary funds. He began calling me, or having his caregiver call, every few days, sobbing and fearful over not having any money to live on. He would routinely forget how or why he had given over money management to me, and seemed not to fully understand how he was supposed to live with no money, checks or credit cards. He was constantly fearful that he would run out of food, lose the ability to pay for his medications, and be tossed out of his condo. Heaven forbid, he might even lose cable! Dad would call, and literally beg me for money, a checkbook or credit cards. It always broke my heart, especially when he would get the answering machine, and leave one of those imploring, and desperate messages. When we did speak, and I always spoke to him about this, he rarely comprehended my explanations.

No matter how hard you try, you will never be able to imagine the number and variety of vultures that descend upon older people and find ways to take their money. On that same trip to Florida, I was appalled at how often the phone rang, and the range of schemes people were proposing. In one exemplary case, after I had steadfastly said no and even hung up several times, the caller became angry, and demanded to know if this was really my father on the phone. When I admitted that is was the son and not the father, he cursed me, threatened me, and even implied that he would be visiting soon to teach me a lesson. I told him he was welcome to try, as that would have been my one opportunity to confront, face to face, one of the bloodsuckers that were bleeding my father dry. He never showed up...but I'll always wonder how much of my father's money this guy had already gotten away with. My father, for his part, had recognized the man's name, admitted he had given him loans and investments, and scolded me for being mean to him. A check with the various agencies in Florida yielded no such name, or business venture.

It pains me to say it, but the charities, even the legitimate ones, weren't much better. They solicited by phone, by mail, in person, every way you can imagine. They solicited early and often, sometimes wanting more money within a month of a contribution. And the more Dad contributed, the more they congratulated him, and the stronger they came on. Now I realize that these people and organizations had no way of evaluating my father's ability to sustain the substantial contributions he was making. I suppose it is asking too much for me to wish that they could have restrained themselves, if even just a bit. But I will say this: they did not have to be so aggressive with their solicitations, nor did they have to be so smoothly persuasive with all their appeals to the big heart of a sweet, aging man. Wouldn't once a year have been often enough? Wouldn't either mail or phone, or in person, have been enough, instead of all three? Couldn't they have held off after a contribution was made, instead of letting Dad know how much more they could do if he could be just a bit more generous?

For years after my father died, I was still getting calls and letters from some of these charities, all of whom found me by tracking him;

none were sent my address as a contact point for my father. In fact, he still gets some of their solicitations here, after years in the grave. Not long ago, one of them called him here. I told the lady that Dad had been dead since 1997, and not kindly, since this had been one of the most aggressive charities. She paused for a brief moment, said she was sorry, and without missing a beat, asked if I would contribute and would agree to be added to their list. I'm still laughing.

I feel strongly that some form of state or federal action is needed to control the rampage of solicitors. Those who are especially dangerous are those offering sweepstakes with entry fees, free giveaways in return for looking over a product or considering an offer, those that supposedly save you money or protect your money, and those free trials which require positive actions to avoid being billed. Seniors, particularly those with diminished capacity, are extremely susceptible to such gimmicky offers, and are not able to discriminate among them, or to make rational choices. Charities, too, should be forced to follow some basic ground rules, before they turn most of our seniors into charity cases themselves.

In the meantime, your aging parent has only one protector: YOU.

What can you do? First and foremost, take away their cash, checks and credit cards, or at least find a way to limit how much money they can go through.

Second, stop their mail, switching their mailing address either to your house, or to a post office box, so that their mail can be screened. Otherwise, have a neighbor or someone else you trust, start getting to the mailbox ahead of them, and screening the mail for you. It is tough to limit access to their mail, as my father and many seniors make picking up the mail, sorting through the magazines/ads/bills/letters/notices, etc., and responding, the highlight of their day. But be prepared, the mail is dangerous! My father was also sending money routinely to two bogus correspondents, believing them to be his mortgage company and stockbroker.

Third, have all the phone calls screened. If he/she has daycare, have that person answer the phone. If not, install an answering machine, keep it on all the time, and then you can at least see who is calling and what they want. You cannot cut off the phone; they need it for emergencies. But you had better get control of how it is used.

What kinds of arrangements and documents will we need?

At the very least you should have:

Power of attorney

Living Will and Health care surrogate

A Legally Binding Will, drafted in the state they live in

Some kind of trust

Power of attorney allows you to sign any and all official documents, and even to make certain financial decisions. It allows you to do business in your father's name, and make binding commitments. Don't do this with computer software, or with anyone but a knowledgeable elder care attorney. Get the broadest powers available under the laws of the state he lives in.

A Living Will and Health Care Surrogate will give you the authority to make decisions about your father's health and well being. This includes treatments, duration of life support procedures, etc. You may not want to think about this, but now is the time to get the authority.

A Legally Binding Will, which again, must be consistent with the laws and practices to the state he lives in. This is not to say that a generic will is useless; it certainly is better than nothing, but you need a proper will, especially if you are not the sole heir. The will must also specify an executor, which can be more than one person, but that is not doing anyone any favors. Funeral preferences, and arrangements for funeral finances should also be in here, as well as provision as to how this will affects, or does not affect, any other financial arrangements, such as trusts.

There are many kinds of trusts, and, contrary to popular belief, trusts are not just for rich people. Trusts can be used to insure that money will be handled consistent with the wishes of the person whose assets are involved; they can be used to streamline the process of transferring assets after death; and they can be used to facilitate the responsible management of your father/mother's assets while he/she is still alive. Trusts can be revocable or irrevocable, which affects the issue of control, but also has implications for things like tax liability and Medicaid eligibility. Consult your attorney. We opted for a living trust, which meant that my father was still alive; made it irrevocable - could not be canceled - and made me the sole trustee. One of the advantages of a living trust is that it can go on in perpetuity, meaning that you can seamlessly use it to manage the assets even after your father has passed away. Assets in the trust do not have to go through probate, which makes it much easier to settle your father's debts and pay his bills, as there will be no period during which you cannot access these resources.

You can make your living parent a trustee, as well as any other relatives or non-relatives. A parent with Alzheimer's is not a good candidate to be a trustee, though one in good shape, might be OK and this in fact, could well be the means to get him/her to agree to set up the trust. We opted for a single trustee for ease of management, but this may not suit all families. My own brother was extremely cooperative, understanding and trusting, which helped immensely. You may not be so lucky; having multiple siblings as trustees can be a nightmare, but if this is the only way to gain everyone's cooperation, it is certainly worth considering. Remember, the size of your father's estate has nothing to do with whether you need to establish a trust; the trust simplifies management of his assets, and gives you broad authority to handle his affairs. Make sure that you move assets into the trust once it is established, as this will consolidate your management task, and gain all the advantages mentioned above for all assets moved. Consult your attorney as to what reasons there might be to retain selected assets outside of the trust...but don't do it by accident. Be sure to structure the trust to make it clear who is in control; otherwise, all may be chaos.

Your living trust, as noted earlier, can be maintained indefinitely as an asset management tool. Your first responsibility will be to insure that, as long as your father is alive, that he is taken care of. This constitutes not only a moral, but also a legal obligation, if the trust is established "for the benefit of" or FBO, your father. Once your father does pass, you must proceed expeditiously to insure that the assets of the trust are distributed to your father's heirs according to the terms of his will, unless the heirs agree to retain their respective shares in the trust, maybe because you are doing such a fabulous job of managing the money. Don't count on it! In any event, they do not relinquish their share of the assets, even if the money stays in the trust for a while. The ideal situation would have you serve as both trustee and executor of the will. You will need to enjoy the confidence of the heirs in order for your job to be as easy as possible...but that may be hard to achieve. It is in their interests to allow you to do your work, unimpeded, if possible, since this will expedite the disposition of assets. If they don't trust you, the job can still be done, but it will take about three to four times as long. The other heirs should remember, as should you, that you are bound by your fiduciary responsibility to administer the trust and estate in accordance with your parent's wishes, no matter how flexible your powers may be. So, don't shrink from that responsibility: if your attorney has done her job, you will have all the authority you need to do what has to be done.

If you don't want the burden of the trust or estate, you can always set up the trust and name a trustee and an executor who your parent respects and the family can have some confidence in. This can be an attorney, accountant, business manager, or a lay person with good business skills. You or any trustee and executor may be compensated for this work, and your attorney can help you set a reasonable rate, whether for you or a designee.

Don't be shy...it is a great deal of work. Set a reasonable rate, and keep track of your time and other expenses.

Chapter Ten

Memory Dies, But Love Endures

Kerhonkson, New York (The Catskills) July 1947: Love Letters

She almost missed the letter. The envelope was not large, but more the size of a smallish greeting card, yet it was the most important piece of mail she had received in her 26 years of life. The letter was from him...he had written, just as he promised, even though she knew it was not something that he did easily, or often. They had only been apart for a few days, but right now the two weeks she had decided to spend with her parents in the mountains seemed as though it would stretch into eternity. Yet, somehow, with the letter she found poking out from under some other mail on the kitchen table, she had a feeling that the remaining time might go faster.

She was not going to read the letter here in the kitchen, for soon she would not be alone. Even here in the Catskills, with summer heat shimmering in through the screens in the open windows, her mother was sure to be in the kitchen by noon, loading huge cast iron pots onto the stove, to begin the massive evening meal. Her father expected that much, and this was one tradition that no amount of New World adaptation could interrupt. With the arrival of her mother, she could also count on a small band of her nieces and nephews, who would trail mother into the kitchen, in eager anticipation of the goodies that their grandmother would find to keep them occupied while she cooked. She did not want to be interrupted, but she also was not prepared to be mean to the little ones, so she knew she must find a private place to read her letter.

She headed out the screen door, pushing it open a bit too eagerly, so that the slam as she sailed through rang out far louder than she had intended. No matter, her mother was not up at the house yet, and her father was hard of hearing to the point of not noticing anything short of a bomb blast. She hurried across the worn grass that dotted the small front yard of their faded wooden bungalow, and dashed past the huge slatted swing that hung lazily from the branch of a huge oak tree. She headed quickly down a small hill to a sweet green spot beside the stream that served as her private picnic spot when she needed to get some peace and quiet. No one usually would approach her here, as they knew she came here to think, read, and sometimes to write poetry.

There were no chairs, but a large flat boulder that had seen the centuries pass at this spot served as the perfect place to sit. She gathered her long skirt under her and folded her slim legs comfortably, for the occasion. The envelope was still in her hand, now a bit warm and even moist, from being held so tightly in her fist as she ran. Carefully, she opened it, not wanting to damage the contents and miss even one word.

Suddenly she caught herself...reflecting upon her own breathless anticipation, and the greedy way in which she hoarded the envelope and its contents. This was not like her, this girlish frenzy over a letter from a boy...well...a man. She was a grown woman, a college graduate, and a professional teacher. For 1947, she was what would later be called a liberated woman, with a ton of self-confidence, a career, and no desire to rush into marriage. Yet, for the first time in her life she found herself all aflutter over a relationship, which was odd, since she had taken four months to even decide that she would drop the other man she had been dating, and see this one on an exclusive basis. But somehow, just now, she was completely mesmerized by the letter in her hand. Maybe this relationship was, in fact, very special.

She opened the letter, and began to read, scanning each paragraph quickly to get the gist, and then re-reading, to be sure she had not

missed anything.
  The letter read as follows:
  Bronx, New York
  July 5, 1947

  My Dearest Darling,
  I tried to wait a whole week to write my first letter, but could stand it no longer after two days, so forgive me if I am writing too soon. Never have I been so lonely, as I am this week, without you. We went to Coney Island for the 4th of July, but even with most of my brothers and their wives, and about a million nieces and nephews to play with, I was miserable without you. I must say, that the only thing that kept me from being utterly inconsolable was knowing that you would return in two weeks time, and that I could see you again.
  I walk the city streets to catch the bus for work in the mornings and I think of you. It has been so hot (is it just as hot up there in the Catskills, or a bit cooler?) that you can almost see the heat rising from the pavement. And as it does, I think of how lucky the heat must be to rise around you, when you walk to the bus, enfolding you as though it were your beau, holding you in its embrace. Then I get on the bus, and pretend that you are sitting next to me, telling me about what you are going to do today and asking me what we should plan for the evening.
  At work, I daydream more than ever. It is so strange to daydream this way. Even through five long years in the Army, through so many boring days when we were well behind the lines and not pressed to do much, I never daydreamed so much. Now, I have you to occupy my mind, and I really don't want to share my thoughts with anyone else, but you. I picture you smiling and telling me an amusing story about one of your students at school, or I picture you so animated, telling me about your plans for the future. I know that you are determined to marry someone with a bright future that you can share, and I keep hoping that you believe that man will be me.

  Sometimes I worry that my plans are too vague...that my moving from job to job since the war makes me look like too much of a wanderer for you. But I will be successful...maybe not rich, but successful. And I know that is all you ask for, for someone with ambition and plans for the future. I WILL be a great inventor someday I swear it. I work on my inventions now, all the time, when I'm not at work, especially since you went up to the mountains. My brother Manny says he knows people in the toy business in New York, and that some of them may be able to help me show my inventions to the people who make decisions at the toy companies. Meanwhile, I am learning the retail business, and sales, and lots of other useful skills. We would not starve...this, I know. My other brother has just gotten a job with a big defense contractor, and they are hungry for qualified electrical engineers, so I might even work there for a time. I know I can make you happy.

I think your teaching makes you very happy, and I envy you. That's why I am more determined than ever to try my hand at inventing. I have been inventing toys since I was a boy, and to see your face light up when you talk about teaching, really motivates me to pursue my passion as well. What a great couple we would make!!

I don't even go out to lunch at work. There is a back room at the store, which they let me use to work on my inventions. Today, I finished carving my two boxers out of soft wood for the boxing figures I am working on. Tomorrow, or maybe tonight, I will attach all the springs to their heads, arms and legs and then will put wires through their hands so they can box. Once finished, two kids will be able to each control one boxer, moving their fingers to throw punches until one knocks the other boxer's head off...well, really the head will just pop up...and that will be a "knockout".

At least when I am working on my inventions, life with you away is tolerable. Walking home from the bus is the worst time, as I keep thinking of what we might be planning for the evening, only to remember that you are so far away. I fool myself into thinking that you are walking next to me, I see your beautiful smile, I see your hair swaying as you walk, I feel your lovely hand in mine, and I even smell your perfume on each warm breeze. Do you think of me? Do you think I am there, or wish I were? Is it beautiful where you are? Never have two days seemed like two years, not even in the army. I long to see you and touch your hand, to smell your perfume. I need to hear your voice and your laugh. I love to watch you laugh...dearest. Please don't think me pathetic, for I am not. This feeling is sad, but not desperate...in fact, it is in many ways...invigorating. Having you in my life, has transformed me...I am a new man. Everything in life now seems to matter more, to be more important. And the future looks like a bright, shimmering path, rather than the murky mush it once appeared to me. I am lonely tonight, but my life is rich and full, thanks to you. Enjoy your vacation and your family, but come back soon, to me, and let me tell you all this, and more, in person.

I Love You...
S-

After reading the letter for the third time, she folded the precious paper back up, slowly, careful not to put any new creases in the thin paper. Never had she known him to be so articulate; perhaps it was easier for him in a letter, or perhaps it was her absence that had inspired him. In any event, she had to see him, of that she was sure. She only had to decide whether to go into town to use the telephone, or to write a letter of her own, but she was going to invite him up for the last weekend they were there. The time was still a week and half away, but she could make it. And the time had come for her parents to realize what she had finally figured out: this was a very special man, and a very special relationship. They would be fine; they already liked him very much, and her mother was eager for more grandchildren. That would have to wait...but maybe a wedding was not too far in her future. After all, he had asked her to marry him on their second date, months ago.

That girl was destined to be my mother.

Fairfax County, Virginia July 1997
My father sat on a sofa just outside the main office of the nursing

home. He was smiling, and his eyes were more focused than usual. He lit up, and I thought he was excited about seeing me, but it was clearly someone just behind me that was the object of his excitement. As I looked back, I could see that ninety-three year old Mrs. McGinty had emerged from the dining room.

The two residents exchanged smiles and hellos, and Mrs. McGinty took my father's outstretched hand. Now he noticed his grandson, David, and me and gave us a warm, though uncertain greeting. I said hello to my Dad, and reminded him who we were this time. He nodded, enthusiastically, and motioned for me to come closer. He still gripped Mrs. McGinty's hand in his.

"Here is your mother, aren't you glad to see her?" His eyes gleamed. At that moment, Susan and Diana joined us. Dad had a smile for them to, as he did for Alan, who came in just a moment later.

I had hailed Mrs. McGinty already, as she was a welcome presence always. But I repeated my hello, and responded to her open arm with a slight hug. We all hugged that dear lady. Dad went on, obviously pleased with himself.

"You know how upset I get when I can't find her. At least I know where she is now. We're going out later to visit our old neighbors from New York who have come to visit. We are taking them to the country club for lunch. Want to come?"

I told Dad that we could not, but wished him a good time. I thought about the life that he and my mother had enjoyed together until she passed away in 1982 at just sixty years old. I thought about how lucky he had been to meet his Annie, who for a time had made him the happiest he had been since my mother died, and how tragic it was for his Alzheimer's to have robbed them of their golden years together. I thought about the depths of his grief and loneliness that had made him see my mother in all the females he had encountered on his journey through dementia, from his in-home caregivers to fellow residents in the nursing home.

I looked at my own family, one so like the one I had grown up with, and hoped that my children would love and revere me the way

I had my father, yet praying that they would not have to nurse me through this kind of agony. My brother met my eye, and cheered me with a slight smile. I was glad he was here.

Susan often said that if you had to wind up in a nursing home that suffering from Alzheimer's or other dementia might well be the way to go. After all, for some time now Dad had been feeling less loneliness, and less confusion. He exhibited fewer and fewer signs of feeling regret or sense of loss. He barely knew what planet he was on, and was content, for the most part, to live in the moment. Maybe that wasn't so bad after all. He was certainly more at peace than the many folks who screamed, or ranted and raved about the injustice of being in this place.

It was terrifying to think that this could happen to me, but we were the only ones feeling sad; Dad no longer knew any regrets or frustration. I realized too that he was probably lucky to have us, his two sons, grandchildren, a daughter-in-law, who all cared and came to see him. We still brought him presents at holiday time, and dined with him when we could. Rarely did we let a week go by without seeing him.

I knew that I needed to get past my disappointment at spending time in this institutional setting. No matter now good an institution it was. There was no way to go on feeling miserable and self-pitying about losing the father I had always known and loved, and railing against the injustice of watching Dad lose his creativity, his genius, even his sense of humor. I did feel lucky to still have him alive, and close by, and to be able to look at him, and hug him. Maybe Susan was right.

Suddenly, the tragedy of it all could not bring me down, for at this moment my Dad was smiling…and feeling no pain.